Chi Kung for
Prostate Health
and Sexual Vigor

Chi Kung
for Prostate Health
and Sexual Vigor

A Handbook of Simple Exercises and Techniques

Mantak Chia
and William U. Wei

Destiny Books
Rochester, Vermont • Toronto, Canada

Destiny Books
One Park Street
Rochester, Vermont 05767
www.DestinyBooks.com

Destiny Books is a division of Inner Traditions International

Originally published in Thailand in 2012 by Universal Tao Publications under the title *Prostate Chi Kung: Techniques and Exercises for Prostate Gland Cancer Prevention and Sexual Vitality*

Library of Congress Cataloging-in-Publication Data
Chia, Mantak, 1944–
  [Prostate chi kung]
  Chi kung for prostate health and sexual vigor : a handbook of simple exercises and techniques / Mantak Chia, William U. Wei.
     pages cm
  "Originally published in Thailand in 2012 by Universal Tao Publications under the title Prostate chi kung : techniques and exercises for prostate gland cancer prevention and sexual vitality"—Provided by publisher.
  Includes bibliographical references and index.
  ISBN 978-1-62055-227-8 (pbk.) — ISBN 978-1-62055-228-5 (e-book)
  1. Qi gong. 2. Sexual health. 3. Generative organs, Male—Diseases—Prevention. I. Wei, William U. II. Title.
  RA781.8.C4693 2013
  613.7'1489—dc23
                                                                2013028933

Printed and bound in the United States

10 9 8 7 6 5

Text design by Priscilla Baker and layout by Virginia Scott Bowman
This book was typeset in Garamond Premier Pro with Present as a display typeface

Illustrations by Udon Jandee
Photographs by Sopitnapa Promnon

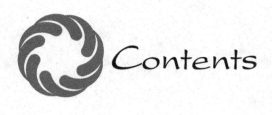

Contents

Acknowledgments

The Universal Tao Publications staff involved in the preparation and production of *Chi Kung for Prostate Health and Sexual Vigor* extend our gratitude to the many generations of Taoist masters who have passed on their special lineage, in the form of an unbroken oral transmission, over thousands of years. We thank Taoist Master I Yun (Yi Eng) for his openness in transmitting the formulas of Taoist Inner Alchemy.

We offer our eternal gratitude to our parents and teachers for their many gifts to us. Remembering them brings joy and satisfaction to our continued efforts in presenting the Universal Healing Tao system. As always, their contribution has been crucial in presenting the concepts and techniques of the Universal Healing Tao.

We wish to thank the thousands of unknown men and women of the Chinese healing arts who developed many of the methods and ideas presented in this book. We offer our gratitude to Bob Zuraw for sharing his kindness, healing techniques, and Taoist understandings.

We thank the many contributors essential to this book's final form: the editorial and production staff at Inner Traditions/Destiny Books for their efforts to clarify the text and produce a handsome new edition of the book and Nancy Yeilding for her line edit of the new edition.

We also wish to thank Colin Drown and Jean Chilton for their editorial work on the earlier edition of this book.

A special thanks goes to our Thai production team: Hirunyathorn Punsan, Saysunee Yongyod, Udon Jandee, and Saniem Chaisam.

Putting Prostate Chi Kung into Practice

The practices described in this book have been used successfully for thousands of years by Taoists trained by personal instruction. Readers should not undertake the practice without receiving personal transmission and training from a certified instructor of the Universal Healing Tao, since certain of these practices, if done improperly, may cause injury or result in health problems. This book is intended to supplement individual training by the Universal Healing Tao and to serve as a reference guide for these practices. Anyone who undertakes these practices on the basis of this book alone, does so entirely at his or her own risk.

The meditations, practices, and techniques described herein are not intended to be used as an alternative or substitute for professional medical treatment and care. If any readers are suffering from illnesses based on mental or emotional disorders, an appropriate professional health care practitioner or therapist should be consulted. Such problems should be corrected before you start training.

Neither the Universal Healing Tao nor its staff and instructors can be responsible for the consequences of any practice or misuse of the information contained in this book. If the reader undertakes any exercise without strictly following the instructions, notes, and warnings, the responsibility must lie solely with the reader.

This book does not attempt to give any medical diagnosis, treatment, prescription, or remedial recommendation in relation to any human disease, ailment, suffering, or physical condition whatsoever.

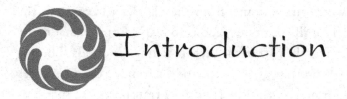

Introduction

After more than fifty years of sharing Prostate Chi Kung daily practice through the Universal Healing Tao system, we find it hard to believe that 70 percent of men over the age of sixty suffer from prostate gland malfunctioning or prostate gland cancer, which can lead ultimately to death. The simple techniques of Prostate Chi Kung enable every man to literally get in touch with his urogenital area and eliminate such problems and discomforts by simply touching himself with the proper intentions. At the suggestion of Ehud Sperling, the publisher of Inner Traditions/Destiny Books, we have gathered together in this book a series of Universal Healing Tao techniques and daily exercises that will support prostate health and sexual vigor. Debilitating urogenital decline is not inevitable for older men. With this simple daily practice, the prostate and urogenital system can function well into advanced old age.

Cancer is the uncontrolled growth of abnormal cells, which feed off the body to maintain this growth. When a cell is damaged or altered without repair to its system, it usually dies. However, cancer cells, also termed malignant cells or tumor cells, proliferate and a mass of cancer cells develops. Many cancers and the abnormal cells that compose the cancer tissue are further identified by the name of the tissue that the cells originate from, such as lung cancer, prostate cancer, or colon cancer. Cancer of the prostate gland, an organ in the male reproductive system, is the most common malignancy in American men and the second leading cause of deaths from cancer, after lung cancer.

The prostate gland is located at the base or outlet (neck) of the urinary bladder. The gland surrounds the first part of the urethra, the passage through which urine drains from the bladder to exit from the penis. One function of the prostate gland is to help control urination by pressing directly against the part of the urethra that it surrounds. The primary function of the prostate gland is to produce some of the substances that are found in normal semen, the fluid that transports the sperm to assist with reproduction.

In a young man, the normal prostate gland is the size of a walnut. During normal aging, however, the gland usually grows larger. This hormone-related enlargement with aging is called benign prostatic hyperplasia (BPH), a condition that is not associated with prostate cancer. However, both BPH and prostate cancer can cause similar problems in older men. An enlarged prostate gland can squeeze or impinge on the outlet of the bladder or the urethra, leading to difficulty with urination. The resulting symptoms commonly include slowing of the urinary stream and urinating more frequently, particularly at night. In addition to causing difficulty with urination, prostate cancer may cause pain, problems during sexual intercourse, or erectile dysfunction.

Prostate cancer tends to develop in men over the age of fifty. Although it is one of the most prevalent types of cancer in men, many never have symptoms, undergo no therapy, and eventually die of other causes, such as heart or circulatory disease, pneumonia, other unconnected cancers, or old age. This is because cancer of the prostate is, in most cases, slow growing and symptom free. However, there are cases of aggressive prostate cancers, in which cancer cells break away from the original mass, travel through the blood and lymph systems, and lodge in other areas, particularly the bones and lymph nodes, where they repeat the uncontrolled growth cycle. This is termed metastatic prostate gland cancer. About two-thirds of cases are slow growing, the other third more aggressive and fast developing.

According to the American Cancer Society, the estimated lifetime risk of being diagnosed with prostate cancer is 17.6 percent for Caucasians and 20.6 percent for African Americans, and the lifetime risk of death is 2.8 percent and 4.7 percent respectively. As reflected by these numbers, prostate cancer is likely to impact the lives of a significant proportion of men alive today. Over the years, however, the death rate from this disease has shown a steady decline because of early detection, and currently more than 2 million men in the United States are still alive after being diagnosed with prostate cancer at some point in their lives. The age and underlying health of the man, the extent of metastasis, and the response of the cancer to initial treatment are important in determining the outcome of the disease.

Cancer can potentially be caused by anything that influences a normal body cell to develop abnormally, such as stagnant energy flow, energy blockage, or improper diet. Some cancer causes remain unknown, while other cancers may develop from more than one known cause. Some may also be developmentally influenced by a person's genetic makeup. Many men develop prostate cancer due to a combination of these factors.

Food and sex are humankind's greatest appetites. From a Taoist's point of view they also offer opportunities for our greatest healing exercises, if we have the proper understanding of how use them to heal our bodies. From the Universal Healing Tao system, as demonstrated in the Destiny Books editions of several Universal Healing Tao publications—particularly *Sexual Reflexology* (prostate gland exercises), *Bone Marrow Nei Kung* (genital massage and Chi Weight Lifting), *Cosmic Detox* (cleansing the front and back doors of the body), and *Cosmic Nutrition* (cancer prevention diet)—we have assembled a sequence of Prostate Chi Kung daily practices that will balance and maintain a healthy prostate gland.

The prostate gland exercises, the genital massage techniques, and Chi Weight Lifting are all aspects of what is known in the Universal Tao system as Bone Marrow Nei Kung. *Nei Kung* means "practicing with your internal power" and Bone Marrow Nei Kung is a Taoist art of self-cultivation that employs mental and physical techniques to rejuvenate the bone marrow, thereby enhancing the blood and nourishing the life-force within.

Bone Marrow Nei Kung overlaps with three primary Taoist approaches to sexual energy: Healing Love, Sexual Energy Massage, and Chi Weight

Lifting. These three methods are used to increase sexual energy and hormones in the body, providing the means to achieve great personal power.

The Healing Love practices enable a person to retain sexual energy, stimulate the brain, and rejuvenate the organs and glands to increase the production of Ching Chi (sexual energy). The techniques reverse the usual outward flow of sexual energy during the orgasmic phase of sex, and draw the Ching Chi upward into the body, thereby enhancing internal healing capabilities. The release of Ching Chi into the body through the Sexual Energy Massage or Chi Weight Lifting methods presupposes that it is already abundant within the sexual center. If one suffers from chronic impotence, weakened kidneys, or any internal dysfunctions, the Healing Love methods should be mastered to accumulate Ching Chi before attempting the other two methods.

In this book, exercises derived from the Healing Love practice are used as nonsexual techniques that help to rejuvenate the internal organs and glands with sexual energy. The Healing Love practices of Testicle Breathing, Scrotal Compression, and the Power Lock can be found in chapter 1, "Prostate Gland Exercises." Also included in chapter 1 are important beginning steps such as cultivating the energy of the five elements through internal organ massage, breathing exercises, and pubococcygeus (PC) muscle exercises.

While Healing Love prevents the loss of Ching Chi and rejuvenates the internal system, the Sexual Energy Massage, presented in chapter 2, releases higher concentrations of Ching Chi into the body for cultivating the bone marrow and stimulating the endocrine glands. When used together, the two practices constitute a safer method of disseminating sexual energy than Chi Weight Lifting. Chapter 2 also includes other forms of genital massage such as the Penis Power Stretching and Penis Milking exercises, and the Cloth Massage.

Chi Weight Lifting, presented in chapter 3, is the ultimate practice for releasing sexual energy into the body. Its practice provides the greatest abundance of Ching Chi for rejuvenating the bone marrow. It also releases maximum quantities of sexual hormones for the stimulation of the pituitary gland to prevent aging. In addition, the technique exercises the fascial connections between the genitals and the internal system, thereby strengthening the organs and glands.

However, Chi Weight Lifting is an advanced practice and should not be attempted without the proper training. After having received Universal Tao instruction, a student may proceed with caution to lift light weights using the genitals. At this level, the Sexual Energy Massage is used before and after Chi Weight Lifting, first to prepare the genitals, and afterward to replenish the circulation in the sexual center, which helps to avoid blood clots. The Healing Love practices that require sexual arousal are no longer necessary because Chi Weight Lifting supplies the body with abundant Ching Chi. Healing Love must still be practiced during sex, however, unless the time is right for procreation.

Prostate health is also supported by proper nutrition and thorough cleansing of the body, especially its "front and back doors." These topics are covered in chapter 4. Chapter 5 offers a summary version of all of the exercises, for your ready reference.

All of these practices will aid you in breaking up any energetic blockages in the pelvic region, opening up the energetic pathways, and preserving optimum prostate gland functioning to an advanced age, thus supporting your ability to urinate properly and rejuvenating your sexual vitality, as well as maintaining your sexual life without discomfort, pain, or malfunction.

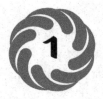

Prostate Gland Exercises

In the East, as well as in the West, exercise is a crucial way to keep the body healthy. But when it comes to increasing sexual energy, the teachers of the East have taken exercise to a new level. To strengthen our sexual energy, and thus strengthen the senses and the whole body, the Eastern traditions have developed exercises that focus specifically on the sexual area. In the Tao, sexual exercises are not merely a way to enhance sexual pleasure or become more attractive. These exercises are a means to enjoy a more vigorous and healthy body, a way to become sensitive to deeper and more intense emotions, and to cultivate spiritual energy.

The sexual area is the root of an individual's health. Leading into the pelvis are a vast number of nerve endings and channels for the veins and arteries. Here are located tissues that communicate with every square inch of the body. All of the major acupuncture meridians that carry energy to the vital organs pass by this area. If it is blocked or weak, energy will dissipate and the organs and brain will suffer. This connectedness is demonstrated by the correspondences detailed in figure 1.1.

Just as the Taoist sexual exercises are designed to charge the brain with energy, increase circulation, and stimulate nerve flow, along with strengthening the urogenital diaphragm and tonifying the energy of the sexual organs, practices that strengthen the internal organs enhance

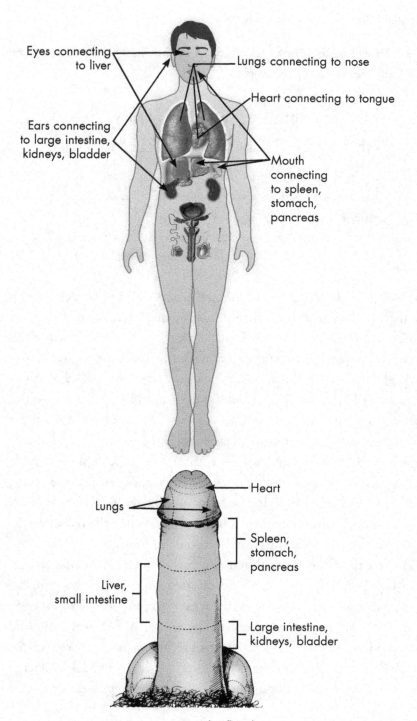

Eyes connecting to liver

Lungs connecting to nose

Heart connecting to tongue

Ears connecting to large intestine, kidneys, bladder

Mouth connecting to spleen, stomach, pancreas

Heart

Lungs

Spleen, stomach, pancreas

Liver, small intestine

Large intestine, kidneys, bladder

Fig. 1.1. Sexual reflexology points

sexual energy. That is why we recommend beginning with basic practices to cultivate the energy of the organs.

INTERNAL ORGANS AND THE ENERGY OF THE FIVE ELEMENTS

The five elemental energies of wood, fire, earth, metal, and water encompass all the myriad phenomena of nature. It is a paradigm that applies equally to humans.

YELLOW EMPEROR'S CLASSIC OF INTERNAL MEDICINE
(SECOND CENTURY BCE)

Sexual prowess, as one aspect of human compatibility and behavior, is derived from the strength of the internal organs. In traditional Chinese medicine, the *internal organs* are much more than the organs themselves. They refer to a quality of energy described in the five elements, five phases of cyclical energetic movement in both nature and in ourselves. For example, the heart is associated with the fire element. The quality of the fire element is expansive, radiant, bright, and warm. The season of the heart is summer, sharing the same qualities of energy.

Each organ is associated with a mental and emotional element as well. So each organ has specific characteristics energetically, physically, emotionally, and spiritually. In the human body, the goal of the Taoist practice is to keep the five elements in harmony. When the five elements are in harmony, the body, mind, and spirit are in balance.

The health of the internal organs greatly affects our sexual energy. Sexual energy is the essence of the internal organs. The body draws the finest energy, especially from the organs, to produce sperm or eggs. When the sexual energy is out of balance, it is reflected in the internal organs, and when one or more organs are out of balance, the sexual energy will definitely be affected. The internal organs and sexual energy are a reflection of each other; when one system is improved, the other follows.

A simple way to draw and spiral sexual energy around the organs is to sit on the edge of a chair, then gently inhale while contracting the penis and drawing the energy up the spine from the penis and out to the organs in the torso (fig. 1.2). The best way to keep the five elements in balance and harmony are the basic Healing Tao practices known as the Inner Smile, Microcosmic Orbit, and Six Healing Sounds. These techniques are presented in chapter 5, "Prostate Chi Kung Summary."

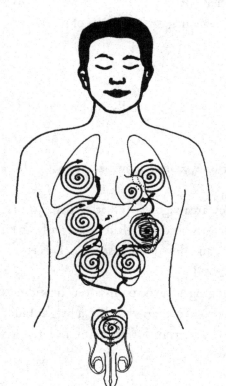

Fig. 1.2. Draw and spiral the energy around the organs.

Massage is another good way to increase energy in the sexual center. It has been used for thousands of years as a way to achieve health, relaxation, and longevity. The reason massage is so beneficial is that it releases pent up tension caused by stress and establishes communication between the mind and body. By increasing circulation, releasing muscle adhesions, and generating positive energy, massage is of utmost importance.

Kidneys and the Water Element

In Taoist medicine, the kidneys, one of the five vital organ systems, are a main source of energy. When they are full of energy, you will be energetic, high-spirited, with plenty of stamina and an abundance of sexual energy. This is all due to the fact that the health of the kidneys is directly related to the health of their corresponding organs, the genitals, and consequently to sexual functioning and capability. The kidneys in Chinese medicine represent the water element in the body. Water is associated with the virtue of gentleness and the negative emotion of fear.

 Kidney Massage

Stimulating and energizing the kidneys is vitally important to healthy sexual energy.

1. Place both hands over the kidneys, on the low back directly above the last rib.
2. Begin to massage the kidney area vigorously with the palms, feeling the heat penetrate deep into the kidneys. Rub vigorously from the lower back, over the kidneys, and down to the sacrum. Feel this entire area open and become energized.
3. After a few minutes of massaging, rest the palms over the kidneys and project energy into the kidneys. You can visualize a bright blue light penetrating into the kidneys and transforming any negative energy into positive.

Knocking or Tapping

Another very beneficial way to stimulate the kidneys is by gently knocking or tapping the lower back area lightly with a loose fist.

1. Locate the kidneys just above the lowest, or floating, rib in the back on either side of the spine. Make a fist and hit the kidneys with the

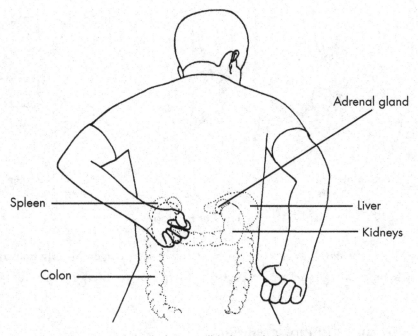

Adrenal gland

Spleen

Liver

Kidneys

Colon

Fig.1.3. Hitting the kidneys will help to shake out sediment.

back of the fist between the wrist and the knuckles (fig. 1.3). Hit only as hard as is comfortable. Knock all the way down to the sacrum and back up to the kidneys, bringing this vibration into the entire lower back area. Do this about 9 times.

2. Alternate hands and sides of the back.
3. Rub your hands together to warm them. Then rub your palms up and down over the kidneys until they feel warm.

 Massage the Ears

The ears, according to traditional Chinese medicine, are an extension of the Kidney energy. One way to stimulate more energy in the kidneys is to massage the ears (see fig. 1.4 on page 12). The ears have more than 120 pressure points; stimulation of them directly activates sexual energy. That is why couples naturally kiss, nibble, and caress each other's ears.

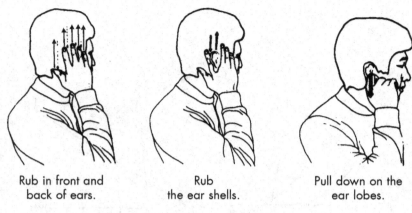

| Rub in front and back of ears. | Rub the ear shells. | Pull down on the ear lobes. |

Fig. 1.4. Ear massage

Place the ear between the thumb and the first finger. Simply massage the whole ear, giving ample pressure to stimulate energy in the entire body.

Heart and the Fire Element

The heart has a strong connection to the sexual center. The heart is associated with the fire element and is the energetic center of passion and affection. It is known as the "king" of all the internal organs, circulating blood and energy through the entire system. The fire element is associated with the virtues of love and joy and with the negative emotions of hatred and cruelty. Negative emotions are elicited when energy is not flowing or when energy is congested in the heart. Have you ever noticed that when you do not communicate what is in your heart and hold in your emotions, there is a feeling of congestion? This is how negative energy is formed. Energy becomes negative when it is not flowing.

Energy stuck in the heart is one of the biggest sexual problems we face. When the energy in the heart is blocked, it is difficult to feel deeply and connect with your partner. For example, when someone in a relationship does not communicate what is in his or her heart, energy is congested and negative emotions ensue. Expressing what is in our hearts in a clear controlled manner frees this energy and transforms it into something positive. It is very healthy to establish the intimate connection between the heart and the sexual center. The Tao regards loving energy and sexual energy as the two strongest energies in the body.

Fire energy is also associated with excitement and exhilaration. It is the fire energy in the heart that opens the sexual center. This is why falling in love leads to sexual desire. Many of the Taoist meditations focus on balancing the heart and sexual center. Even the higher-level Taoist meditations called Kan and Li (Fire and Water) work on unifying these two energies and steaming their potent force through all the energy meridians.

Massage the Chest to Open the Heart

Massage the chest with the fingers or knuckles (fig. 1.5). The knuckles work well for deeper pressure.

1. Look for tender areas along the sternum and between the ribs along the chest. Press into them gently, massaging until you feel a release.
2. It is especially good to spend time massaging the sternum, releasing emotional energy that has congested in the heart center.
3. To end, place the hands over the chest and project energy into the

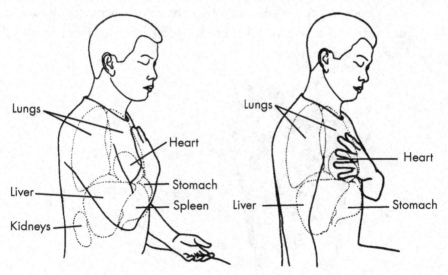

Fig. 1.5. Place the palm on the chest to open the heart.

heart area. Visualize a warm, bright red glow in the heart. Feel the connection between the heart and the sexual center.

Tongue Chi Kung

The tongue is the sense organ of the fire element and the energetic extension of the heart (fig. 1.6). Exercising the tongue is a great way to open the heart and the sexual energy. There is a very strong connection between the tongue, heart, and sexual center. This is why lovers kiss with the tongue. In some cultures kissing with the tongue is just as intimate as making love.

1. To exercise the tongue, bring the tip of the tongue in front of the upper teeth inside the lips. Circle the tongue down to the inside lower lip.
2. Continue to circle in front of the teeth and inside the lips about 36 times and then switch directions.
3. Next, massage the flat part of the tongue against the upper palate vigorously. Feel the heat that is generated through the head and the whole body. Heat is a good sign that the fire element is activated in the heart and sexual center. Massage the tongue against the upper palate at least 36 times.

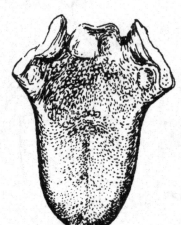

Fig. 1.6. The tongue

Lungs and the Metal Element

The lungs are the organs of breath, keeping us intimately connected to the universe. When inhaling we take in the body of the universe and when exhaling we give back part of ourselves to the universe. The breath is a metaphor of this dynamic exchange of energy. It represents giving and receiving, ebb and flow, male and female. Simply by observing the dynamics of the breath we can witness the balance of yin and yang* and the constant flow and exchange of life-force energy within the universe. Male and female relationships are part of this universal exchange, creating harmony and balance in all apparent opposites.

Our breathing patterns always reflect how we feel. When we become sexually aroused the breath becomes deep and full, pumping energy through the whole body. If the lung energy is weak or congested, it is difficult to feel aroused and excited. The negative energy of the lungs is depression. Depression is one of the biggest causes of impotence and low sexual energy. On the other hand, when energy is flowing in the lungs, we have a feeling of courage and self-expression. Positive energy in the lungs allows you to breathe in life, to experience it. To feel sexually aroused, the whole body needs to be alive and full of energy. This is what the lungs do when they are healthy and full of energy.

Massage the Lung Points

Stimulate and open the lungs by lightly knocking on the chest with a loose fist. This opens the rib cage and relaxes the diaphragm.

1. Knock just below the collar bone to activate the lung points and to stimulate the Lung meridian.
2. Continue to knock on and across the chest for at least 1 minute with both hands.

---

*Yin is analogous to the negative charge, and represents a cool, gentle energy often associated with femininity. *Yang* is the positive charge, and represents a hot, volatile energy that is characteristic of masculinity.

3. Afterward, feel the buzzing and tingling in the chest area. Take 2 or 3 long deep breaths. Feel the lungs open and energize.

Liver and the Wood Element

The liver transfers a tremendous amount of energy to the sexual center. The liver is associated with the wood element and the virtues of kindness and forgiveness. The negative emotions of the liver are frustration (sexual frustration) and anger. When the Liver energy is congested, we simply cannot relax. Relaxation is an indispensable quality of good sexual health. When we are tense and tight, energy does not flow.

The wood element plays a vital role in the strength of the erection for men. When the wood energy is blocked, men usually have a difficult time getting an erection, even though they may feel aroused. Deep relaxation usually solves this problem. Releasing the congestion in the liver allows the wood energy to flow into the sexual center.

Massage the Feet

The Liver meridian runs down the legs and into the feet. Massaging the feet is a great way to relax the body and stimulate the wood element. Whenever the body is able to relax more deeply, the sexual center benefits. When the body is under stress and tight, the sexual energy is constricted.

1. Massage the feet with both hands. Pay particular attention to the big toe. This is where the Liver meridian ends.
2. Spend at least 5 minutes on each foot to ensure that the energy moves into the body.

Spleen and the Earth Element

The spleen is associated with the earth element and the virtues of balance and openness. The negative emotions associated with the spleen are worry and anxiety. When the earth element is out of balance, the feelings of the body are disconnected, making it difficult to get in touch with sensation. For example, when the energy of the spleen is congested, it causes the mind to be overactive. The overactivity in the mind is what causes worry and anxiety. When there is excess energy in the head, it is hard to be in touch with the body.

When energy is flowing in the earth element, we are able to feel our center and our connections to all life. When we feel connected to ourselves, we are able to connect to others, both sexually and emotionally. The abdomen is the center of the body. When the abdomen is full of energy, the body is full of energy.

Massage the Abdomen

1. Massage the abdomen in a gentle circle, rubbing with the flow of digestion, from left to right (fig. 1.7). Continue to circle the hands around the abdomen at least 36 times.
2. With the fingertips, feel for any tightness or congestion. Work into the abdomen and feel the release of tightness.
3. Work with your breathing while you are massaging. See if you can breathe all the way into the belly. Remember, the organs provide energy to the sexual center. When the energy in the abdominal area is full, the sexual center is balanced and harmonized.

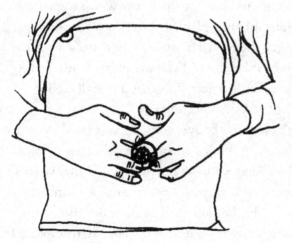

Fig. 1.7. The major key to maintaining good health is to eliminate tension, worry, and toxins every day and maintain good sexual energy by massaging the abdomen.

PROSTATE BREATHING CHI KUNG

There is one way of breathing that is shameful and con-
stricted. Then there's another way: a breath of love that
takes you all the way to infinity.

RUMI, *OPEN SECRET* (TRANSLATED
BY JOHN MOYNE AND COLEMAN BARKS)

The first step to becoming a more sexually powerful person is to learn how to breathe properly. Many of the sexual exercises require a certain level of breath control and when you learn to breathe properly the exercises become much easier and much more powerful.

Breathing exercises are a direct way to control stress. This will be clear if you think about how you breathe when you are in a terribly stressful situation. The breath gets jammed up in the chest in short shallow gasps that barely allow oxygen into the lungs. Under extreme circumstances the breath might become almost nonexistent. With this type of breathing, life-enhancing oxygen does not flow freely through the body. This creates stress and tension, lodging it in the body rather than allowing it to be processed and released.

Long ago in Chinese medicine it was discovered that the breath is a direct reflection of the emotional state of the body. When someone is sad, he or she breathes in short inhaling gasps, locking the air in the upper chest. When someone is angry, the breath is usually long contracted exhalations, with desperately short inhalations. Even when we are not feeling very emotional, the breath will still reflect the general overall feelings in the body, which are often not very empowering.

Just as correct diet enhances the body's store of nutritional essence, so correct breathing enhances the body's supply of vital energy. Proper breathing is performed by the diaphragm, not the rib cage and the clavicles. Because of laziness, ignorance, smoking, pollution, constipation, and other factors, adults these days invariably become shallow chest breathers, rather than the deep abdominal breathers that we are meant to be. All true martial arts and meditation practices use the breath as the gate to control the body.

Breathing abdominally is the most natural thing, but we have forgotten how we used to breathe. Have you ever watched a baby breathe? If not, the next time you have an opportunity, do so. Pay particular attention to how the abdomen does the breathing, not the chest. This is the natural way, the way we must return to.

Chest breathing employs the intercostal muscles between the ribs to forcibly expand the upper rib cage, thereby lowering air pressure in the chest so that air enters by suction. However, this leaves the lower lungs, which contain by far the greatest surface area, immobilized. So about three times as many chest breaths are needed to get the same quantity of air into the lungs as provided by a single diaphragmatic breath.

Deep Abdominal Breathing

A complete, deep abdominal breath should employ three areas of the lungs in a smooth, unbroken expansion that begins at the bottom in the abdomen and not in the upper chest (see fig. 1.8 on page 20).

1. Inhale air slowly into the lower lungs by letting the diaphragm expand and balloon downward into the abdominal cavity. When the diaphragm is fully expanded, the intercostal muscles come into play to open the rib cage and fill the middle lungs with air.
2. As the rib cage reaches full expansion, lift up the clavicles so that air flows into the narrow upper pockets of the lungs.
3. Exhale in the reverse manner, releasing air from the upper part of the chest, downward through the ribs, finally expelling the air out the lower lungs by slightly contracting the abdomen.

Breathing with the diaphragm in this manner reduces the number of breaths per minute by more than half, greatly enhances respiratory efficiency, saves the heart from strain, and conserves vital energy. When we are able to breathe in this manner, the body automatically takes it as a sign to be relaxed and calm. This is one of the best ways to combat the stress of everyday life. If you can, practice deep abdominal breathing whenever

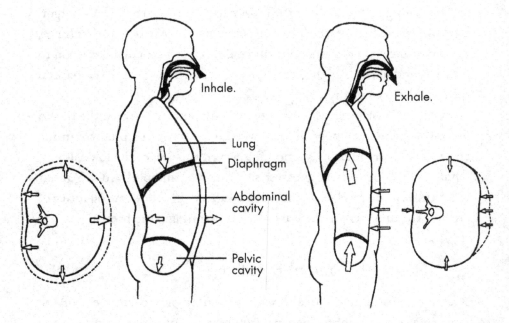

Inhale.

Exhale.

Lung

Diaphragm

Abdominal cavity

Pelvic cavity

Fig. 1.8. Deep abdominal breathing

you have a few extra minutes, driving the car, standing in line, waiting for the dentist, or anywhere else you can imagine; great benefits will result. Pretty soon, with practice, your body will automatically start breathing more deeply subconsciously.

Deep abdominal breathing activates the cranial and sacral pumps and keeps the spinal cord fluid moving in the joints and cranium. Spinal cord fluid and seminal fluid are very similar in nature.

And deep abdominal breathing is a wonderful exercise for increasing sexual energy. It sends energy down through the urogenital diaphragm, loosening and relaxing the whole pelvic cavity. Without deep breathing, the lower abdomen has a tendency to become tight and contracted. With this tightness in the abdomen there is inevitably an imbalance throughout the sexual area. This leads to either low sexual energy or uncontrollable sexual energy. For men, tightness can cause premature ejaculation, wet dreams, impotence, or sexual frustration.

Energizer Breathing

The energy breath is performed by rapidly expelling air out of the lungs and is designed to create efficient circulation, strengthening the energy of the lower abdominal area. Imagine that there is a small fire right behind the navel. To turn this small spark into a vibrant fire air is needed. As you perform the exercise, the breath should sound like a bellows, fanning a fire.

1. Start by forcefully expelling all air from the lungs with a strong contraction of the abdominal wall.
2. Immediately after the expulsion of air, let the lungs fill naturally without effort, about half way.
3. When the lungs are half full, immediately contract the abdominal wall again to forcefully expel another gust of air. The exercise should consist of about 20–30 rapid expulsions of air. This strengthens and energizes the lower abdominal area.

 Testicle Breathing

Testicle Breathing (see fig. 1.9 on page 22) can be practiced sitting, standing, or lying down.

Sitting: Sit on a chair so that your weight is distributed to your legs and buttocks. Cover your genitals with comfortable underwear or loose clothing. Your feet should be flat on the floor and your palms on your knees.

Standing: Stand up straight and relaxed with feet shoulder-width apart and your hands at your sides.

Lying on right side: Use a pillow to raise your head 3–4 inches. Place your right thumb behind your ear and fold it slightly forward; keep the other fingers in front of the ear. Rest your left hand on the outer left thigh. Bend the left knee slightly and rest it on top of the right leg, which should be straight.

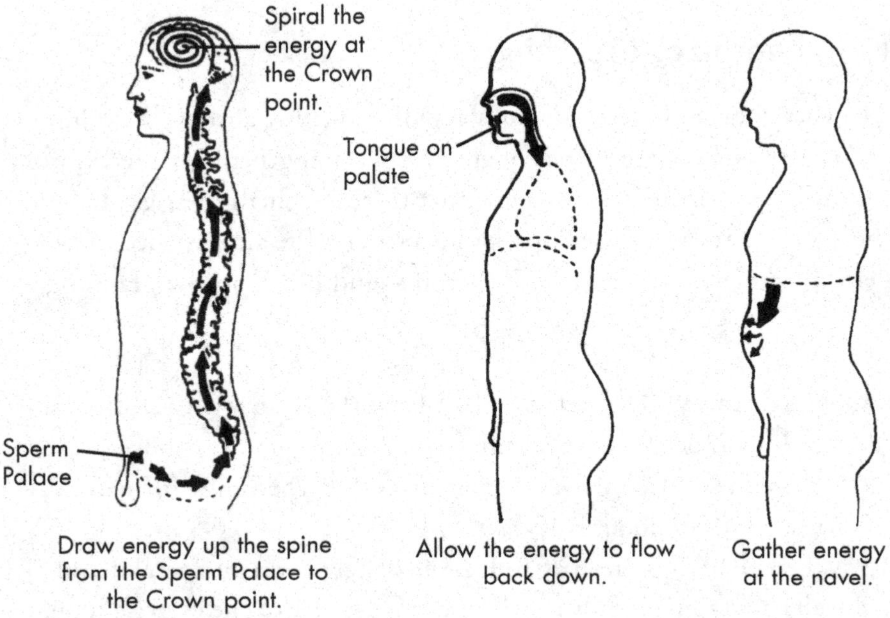

Spiral the
energy at
the Crown
point.

Tongue on
palate

Sperm
Palace

Draw energy up the spine
from the Sperm Palace to
the Crown point.

Allow the energy to flow
back down.

Gather energy
at the navel.

Fig. 1.9. Testicle Breathing

1. Round your neck and shoulders slightly, and place your tongue on the roof of your mouth. Inhalations during this practice should be small sips of air; there may be many inhalations for each exhalation.

2. Inhale through your nose and pull the testicles up. Hold and exhale slowly, lowering your testicles and feeling cool energy in the scrotum. Repeat 9 times.

3. Inhale and pull the energy up to the Sperm Palace at the pubic bone, hold, then exhale slowly. Repeat 9 times.

4. Guide the energy up the back as if sipping on a straw. Press the lower back outward as if flattening it against a wall to activate the sacral and cranial pumps. Hold attention on the sacrum and exhale slowly.

5. Relax sacrum and neck.

6. Inhale and guide the energy up to T11 thoracic vertebrae, and then relax and exhale.

7. Inhale and guide the energy up to the Jade Pillow at the base of the skull, and then relax and exhale.

8. On the final inhalation, guide the energy up to the crown. At the

Crown point, spiral the energy in your brain 9–36 times clockwise, then 9–36 times counterclockwise.

9. After spiraling at the Crown point, place your tongue on your palate and allow the energy to flow down to the third eye, tongue, throat, and heart. Pause for a while at the heart and feel the sexual (creative) energy transform into loving energy, and then move down to the solar plexus and the navel. Collect the energy at the navel.

 ## Scrotal Compression

This exercise dynamically builds sexual power by packing electromagnetically charged energy into the testicles. As an expanding sensation fills the genitals, sexual energy increases, eventually reaching into higher centers of the body through the Microcosmic Orbit. The Microcosmic Orbit runs from the sexual center up the spine to the crown, then down the front of the body and back to the navel. (See chapter 5 for instructions on opening the Microcosmic Orbit.) This practice is particularly important to use after the Sexual Energy Massage (see chapter 2) or Chi Weight Lifting (see chapter 3) to replenish the energy extracted from the genitals.

Warning: Do not engage in these practices if you have any venereal infections or skin rashes in the genital area. The methods used to draw sexual energy into the body can spread existing venereal diseases to the organs.

1. Sit on the edge of a chair with testicles hanging loose over the edge or practice in a standing position.
2. Inhale deeply, expanding the solar plexus, while contracting the anus and pulling energy into the upper abdomen.
3. Compress the energy into a sphere at the solar plexus point (see fig. 1.10 on page 24). Roll this chi ball down the front of the abdomen to the navel, and then down to the pelvic region.
4. Contract the abdominal muscles downward and pack and compress chi into the scrotum for as long as you can. Squeeze the anus and tighten the perineum to prevent energy loss.

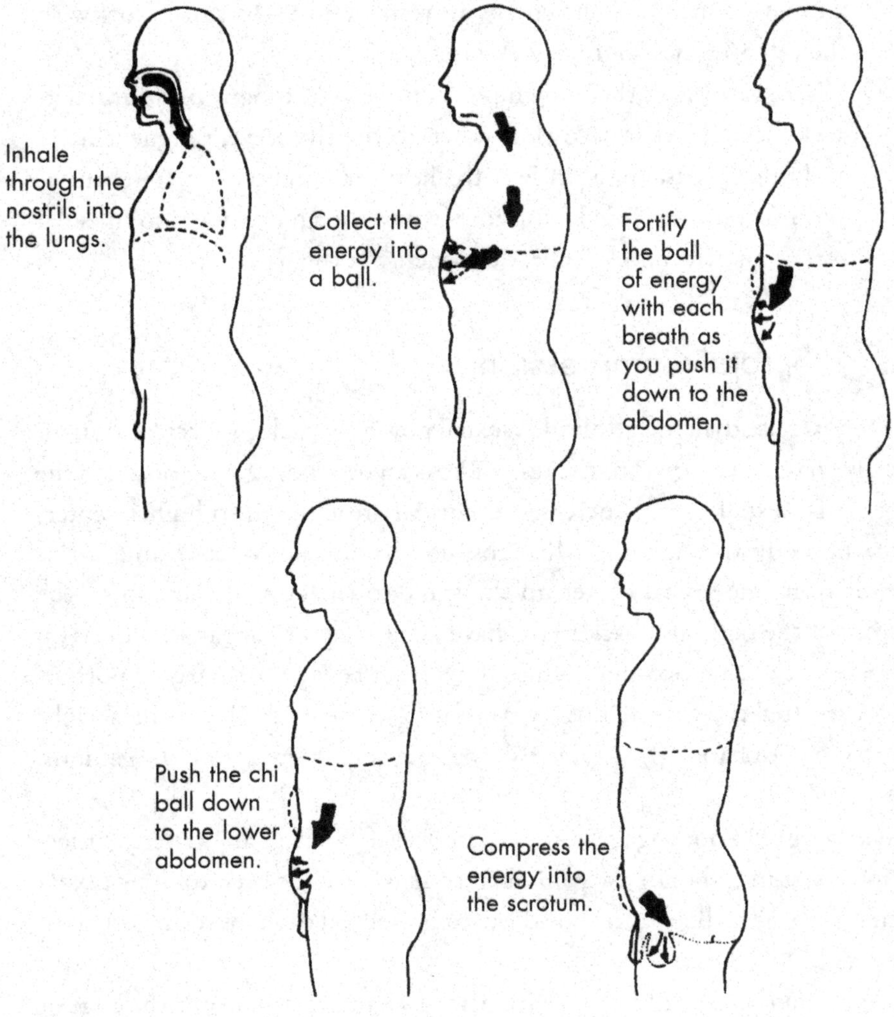

Inhale through the nostrils into the lungs.

Collect the energy into a ball.

Fortify the ball of energy with each breath as you push it down to the abdomen.

Push the chi ball down to the lower abdomen.

Compress the energy into the scrotum.

Fig. 1.10. Scrotal Compression

5. While maintaining the compression, keep your tongue pressed against your palate to maintain energy flow in the Microcosmic Orbit. Swallow deeply into the sexual center.

6. Exhale. Take a few quick short breaths by pulling your lower abdomen in and pushing it out (Energizer Breathing) until you can breathe normally. Relax completely.

7. Repeat the exercise from 3 to 9 times until you feel the testicles become warm.

CULTIVATING SEXUAL ENERGY THROUGH CONTROLLING EJACULATION

In the Taoist view of sexual health, it is important to cultivate our sexual energy rather than needlessly wasting it. For men, this means regulating and controlling ejaculation. Ejaculating too often depletes the source of vital energy, not allowing the water of life to spread to the rest of the body. All schools of Taoism agree that semen retention and proper regulation of its emission are indispensable skills for male adepts. This retention, however, is dramatically different from the religious idea of celibacy. In the Tao, regulating and managing ejaculation does not mean becoming a celibate.

The basic purpose of the Taoist cultivation methods is to increase, as much as possible, the quantity of the life-giving, age-retarding hormones secreted in a man's body during sexual excitement, while at the same time decreasing, as much as possible, the loss of semen and its related hormones through ejaculation.

Exercising Your PC Muscle

Exercising your pubococcygeus (PC) muscle will enable you to develop ejaculatory control, which will prevent the premature urge to ejaculate (see fig. 1.11 on page 26). You will also improve urinary flow and increase blood circulation for enhanced size and sensation, as well as improve sexual stamina, and the ability to have multiple orgasms. These exercises can help save your life by giving you a well-developed, healthy prostate.

The first step to beginning a PC workout is locating your PC muscle. Some men have been able to locate their PC muscle for years without knowing it. If you can make your penis move on its own when you have an erection, you have located your PC muscle. If you cannot do this, the next time you urinate, stop the flow of urine before you finish. The muscle you use to stop yourself from urinating is the PC muscle.

Try doing 10 to 20 flexes of your PC muscle to see how well you can

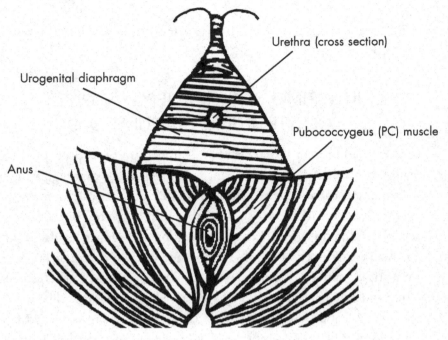

Urethra (cross section)

Urogenital diaphragm

Pubococcygeus (PC) muscle

Anus

Fig. 1.11. Male pelvic floor showing the location
of the pubococcygeus muscle

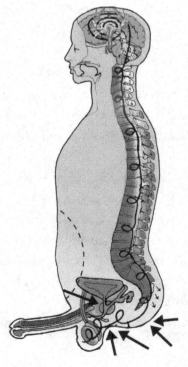

Fig. 1.12. PC muscle
squeezing

focus on them. If your PC feels tired after 20 flexes, you are very out of shape. After you do about 20 or so, flex and squeeze really tight and hold it for as long as you can (see fig. 1.12 on page 26). Ancient Taoists called this exercise "tightening the anus" because flexing the PC muscle also makes your anus tight. Though this may be intimidating at first due to the lack of PC strength, within a few months of continual exercise, you will be able to hold off the urge to ejaculate just by squeezing the PC muscle as tight as you can until the urge goes away.

Your ejaculatory strength and ability, your erectile strength and firmness, and your prostate health and wellness are all directly influenced by how much you perform these PC exercises. You can aim for at least 200 to 500 PC flexes a day.

PC Muscle Exercises

◉ *Warming Up*

1. Start out by squeezing and relaxing your PC muscle at a steady pace for a good 30 flexes.
2. At the end of the set, rest for 30 seconds.
3. Continue with 2 more sets, resting for 30 seconds between each set.

After completing 3 sets, you should have better control over your PC muscle due to the increased flow of blood and chi.

◉ *PC Clamps*

1. Squeeze and release over and over again. Start with sets of 30 and build yourself up to sets of 100 or more.
2. Make sure you do at least 300 PC clamps a day for the rest of your life.

The PC muscle heals quite quickly; you may find yourself waking up with a hard erection every morning. You will soon find that doing this exercise every day is the best move you could ever make for your sexual health and vitality.

Long Slow Squeeze

1. Warm up with a set of 30 clamps, then flex as hard and as deep as you possibly can.
2. When you cannot squeeze any deeper, hold where you are for a count of 20.
3. Rest for 30 seconds.
4. Repeat 5 times.

After a month or so of exercising, you should be able to do squeeze-and-hold sessions for at least several minutes at a time. This particular exercise will give you erections of steel and the ability to last as long as you want in bed. You should eventually work your way up to 10 sets of 2-minute-long holds.

Testicle Stretching Exercise

1. Warm up as you did for the PC exercises.
2. Grasp around the testicles with one hand and the penis with the other and begin stretching them in opposite directions, up and down; at the same time, exhale while flattening the stomach and sticking out the tongue (fig. 1.13). Stop when you feel a good stretch; hold for 20 seconds.
3. After the 20 seconds, relax for a few seconds and grasp around your testicles and penis again.
4. Stretch again, this time pulling your testicles to the left and your penis to your right. Feel a good stretch and hold for 20 seconds. Rest for 10 seconds.
5. Stretch again, this time pulling your testicles to the right and your penis to your left. Wait until you feel a good stretch and hold for 20 seconds. Rest for 10 seconds.
6. Stretch again, this time pulling your testicles down and your penis up. Wait until you feel a good stretch and hold for 30 seconds.

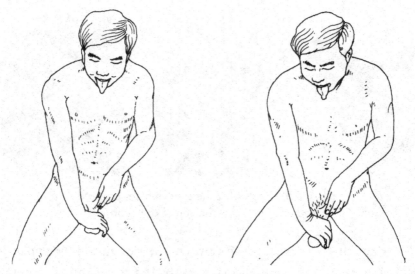

Fig. 1.13. Testicle Stretching

Sexual Energy and the Brain

The Taoist sage says, "Return the sexual energy to revitalize the brain." The sexual organs have a close connection to the center of the brain, especially the pineal gland (fig. 1.14).

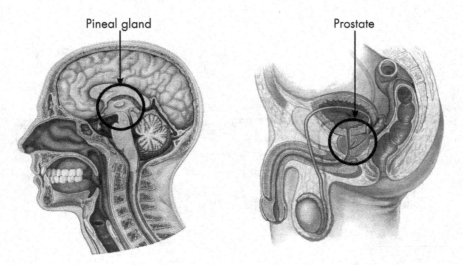

Fig. 1.14. Center of the brain connects to the sexual organs.

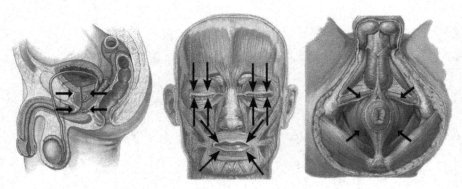

Fig. 1.15. Contracting the eyes, mouth, prostate,
and anus activates the center of the brain.

Circulating the sexual energy down to the sacrum and then up to the brain will increase the brain memory. As you flex the PC muscle, contract the eyes, mouth, anus, and prostate gland to activate the center of the brain (fig. 1.15).

By drawing the sexual energy up to the brain you are changing the physical (sperm) to etheric and the material to immaterial (fig. 1.16). The pineal gland is the second sexual organ. In men the pineal is the female sexual organ (fig. 1.17).

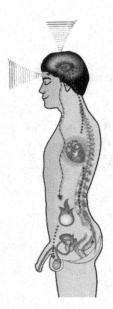

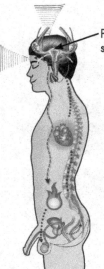

Pineal as female
sexual organ

Fig. 1.16. Changing
the physical to the
etheric by drawing
sexual energy up to
the brain

Fig. 1.17. The
pineal gland is
the female sexual
organ in men.

◯ *Visualize as You Exercise*

1. Close your eyes and get a good picture of your sexual organs in your mind as you exercise.
2. Visualize the Microcosmic Orbit movement and fill the internal organs with chi (see page 126 for Microcosmic Orbit directions).
3. Every time you do a PC flex (or the genital exercises given in the next chapter), visualize your penis and pineal gland growing a little bit and becoming the size that you desire.
4. Focus on every flex, stroke, and stretch, simultaneously visualizing its effect.

The more you make visualization a regular part of your sexual energy workouts, the faster and better results you will attain. This is true for any of the Taoist practices, whether penile fitness, exercise, body conditioning, or meditation. The more you foresee your results and the more you focus on where you want to be, the faster you will get there. Take care and always remember to visualize your goals.

POWER LOCK EXERCISE

The Power Lock should be practiced before and after the Sexual Energy Massage (presented in chapter 2) to assist in the upward draw of released energy and sexual hormones from the perineum to the crown. Air is inhaled through the nose in nine sips as the genitals, perineum, and anus are simultaneously contracted to draw Ching Chi upward. In conjunction with these contractions, the three middle fingers of either hand are applied to a point at the back of the perineum, near the anus (see fig. 1.18 on page 32).

How to Apply the Pressure

Fingernails should be cut short and filed. Using either hand, combine the three middle fingers into a triangle. Immediately after each inhalation, press the three fingertips on the point in front of the anus to lock

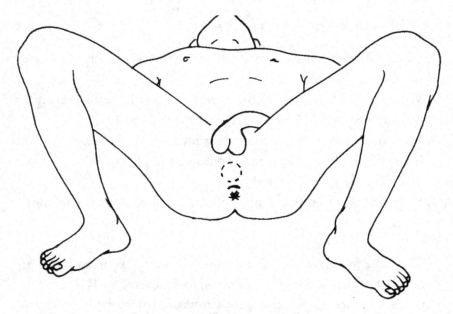

Fig. 1.18. Locate the Gate of Death and Life (the perineum, or Hui Yin) between the sex organ and the anus.

the Ching Chi into its upward journey, preventing its return to the perineum (fig. 1.19). Release the fingertips as you sip in more air and then reapply them as each breath is held. Press the point only for as long as you hold each breath and muscular contraction, then release. Do not apply the fingers as you inhale because you will block the energy from rising. Remember that the fingers help to push the energy upward.

Warning: Before you begin drawing Ching Chi up to the higher centers, remember that you should never leave hot sexual energy in the head for long periods of time. Always draw it down to the navel through the Functional Channel (front) of the Microcosmic Orbit at the end of your practice. There is an old Chinese saying: "Don't cook your brain." When in doubt about the hot or cold status of your energy, store it in the navel.

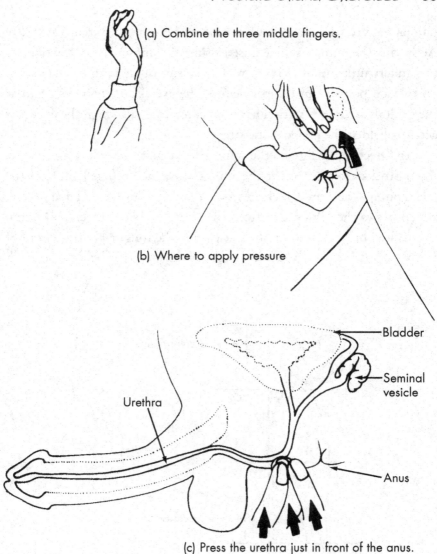

(a) Combine the three middle fingers.

(b) Where to apply pressure

Bladder

Seminal vesicle

Urethra

Anus

(c) Press the urethra just in front of the anus.

Fig. 1.19. The external blocking procedure involves pressing the urethra from a point at the back of the perineum, near the anus.

Activating the Pumps at the Five Stations

The pressure at the perineum helps to guide the rising energy up to five stations: the sacrum, T11, C7, base of the skull, and the crown. Each of the five stations has a "pump" to move energy, but the sacral and cranial pumps require the most concentration to become activated (fig. 1.20). Activating the pumps is done in sets using nine muscular contractions of the undertrunk simultaneously with nine sips of air to draw the energy up to each point from the perineum. The exercise then starts again at the genitals after each station has been completed, although the energy is actually held at the previous station.

To direct the energy up the spine, tilt the sacrum slightly and clench the buttocks as you contract the anus and perineum (fig. 1.21a). As the sacral pump is activated, it creates a vacuum in the urogenital diaphragm, which draws the Ching Chi from the sexual center. The cranial pump is activated by first pressing the flat part of the tongue up to the roof of the mouth as the tip of the tongue presses the lower jaw behind the teeth

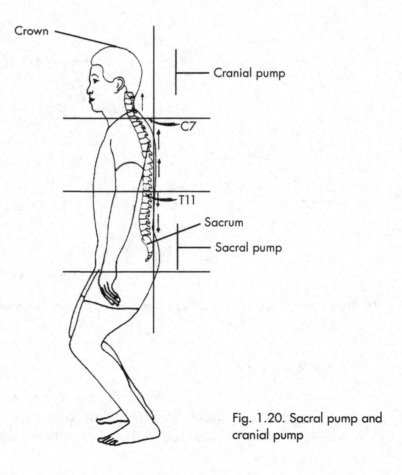

Fig. 1.20. Sacral pump and cranial pump

(fig. 1.21b). Your teeth should be slightly clenched as you pull in the chin toward the back of the head. Take in 10 percent of your lung capacity with each sip of air through your nose as you pull up the genitalia, apply pressure with the three fingers, and contract the individual sections of the undertrunk. Simultaneously push up your tongue, pull in your eyes, and look up to your crown.

Note: Remember never to contract the chest muscles. This can cause energy to congest around the area of the heart.

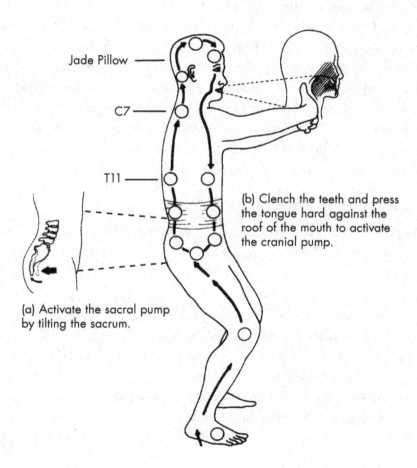

Jade Pillow

C7

T11

(b) Clench the teeth and press the tongue hard against the roof of the mouth to activate the cranial pump.

(a) Activate the sacral pump by tilting the sacrum.

Fig. 1.21. Activating the cranial and sacral pumps

Sequence

After drawing sexual energy from the genitals into the perineum through Testicle Breathing, use a short inhalation to draw the energy through each successive point leading up to the first station. Remember to apply the fingers as you hold each sip of air. First inhale and contract the perineum. Then inhale again as you contract the anus. With the next sip of air, pull up the back part of the anus as you draw the energy up to the sacrum. After covering these points, use several sets of nine contractions to push the energy into the sacrum. This entire sequence is repeated for each subsequent station, starting at the sexual center.

As Ching Chi expands in the sexual center, use one sip of air with each contraction to draw it up through the aforementioned points. At least one set of nine contractions should be used for each station that was previously opened. Then emphasize each new station with several sets of nine contractions. Although a week or two may be required to open each station completely, you can practice using all of the stations, concentrating more on the difficult points. Exhale after the ninth sip of air, and release the tension as you repeat the process.

Four Levels of Power Lock Practice

As you become more experienced in the practice, the upward movement of energy is gradually assured more by mental control than physical control.

1. **Beginners:** Use all muscles and three-finger technique.
2. **Intermediate:** Use fewer muscles and no finger technique.
3. **Advanced:** Use less muscle in perineum and use sacral and cranial pumps more; use more mind control.
4. **Most Advanced:** Pure mind control used to command the penis and move Ching Chi up and down.

Power Lock Practice Step by Step

 ## Station One—the Sacrum

1. Be aware of the sexual organ.
2. When you feel the Ching Chi expanding, inhale and contract the perineum, drawing sexual energy into the perineum. Use your fingers to press on the point each time you contract, releasing them briefly before each subsequent contraction.
3. Inhale, contract the anus, and draw the energy up to the anus.
4. Inhale, contract, and draw the energy up to the back part of the anus.
5. Inhale, and tilt the sacrum as you clench the buttocks to activate the sacral pump. Draw the energy up to the sacrum.
6. Use 9 contractions with 9 sips of air to draw Ching Chi from the sexual center to the sacrum (fig. 1.22).

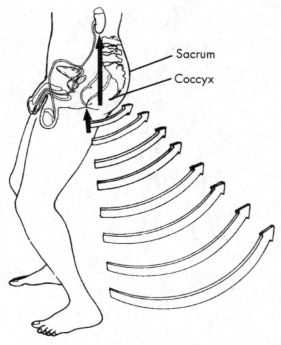

Fig. 1.22. Collect the energy at the sexual center;
then do 9 contractions to draw the energy to the sacrum.

7. Hold the energy at the sacrum as you exhale and return your attention to the sexual organ.

☯ *Station Two—the T11 Point*

1. Repeat the previous steps, drawing the energy up through the sacrum until you reach the T11 point (fig. 1.23).
2. Use 9 contractions with 9 sips of air to draw the Ching Chi from the sexual center to T11 on the spine. (Activate the T11 pump by pushing the spine outward at that point.)
3. Hold the energy there as you exhale and return your attention to the sexual organ.

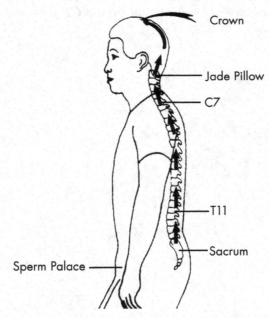

Fig. 1.23. Power Lock: guiding
the energy up to the crown

☯ *Station Three—the C7 Point*

1. Repeat the previous steps, drawing the energy up through T11 until you reach the C7 point (see fig. 1.23).
2. Use 9 contractions with 9 sips of air to draw Ching Chi from the sexual center to the C7 point. (Push the C7 out, and pull back the chin slightly to help activate the C7 pump.)
3. Hold the energy there as you exhale and return your attention to the sexual organ.

☯ *Station Four—the Base of the Skull*

1. Repeat the previous steps, drawing the energy up through C7 until you reach the base of the skull.
2. Use 9 contractions with 9 sips of air to draw Ching Chi from the sexual center to the base of the skull as you activate the cranial pump. Pull the chin back once again (fig. 1.24).

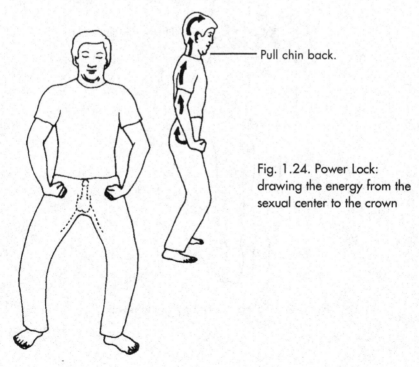

Pull chin back.

Fig. 1.24. Power Lock: drawing the energy from the sexual center to the crown

3. Hold the energy there as you exhale and return your attention to the sexual organ.

⚡ *Station Five—the Crown*

1. Repeat the previous steps, drawing the energy up through the base of the skull until you reach the Crown point (see fig. 1.23 on page 38).
2. Use 9 contractions with 9 sips of air to draw Ching Chi from the sexual center to the crown.

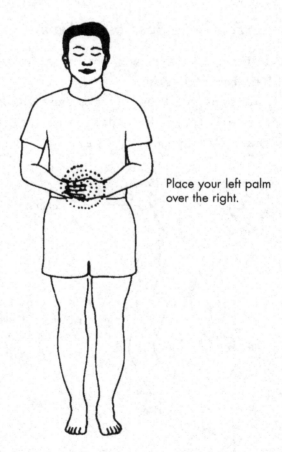

Place your left palm over the right.

Fig. 1.25. Collect the energy at the navel.

3. Exhale and rest as you spiral this energy 9 times outward from the crown, and then 9 times inward.

4. Finally, bring the energy down and store it in the navel.

◎ Completion of the Power Lock

Cover your navel with both palms, left hand over right. Collect and mentally spiral the energy outwardly at the navel 36 times clockwise and then inwardly 24 times counterclockwise (fig. 1.25).

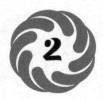

Genital Massage

Taoists regard sexual energy as having creative and rejuvenating powers. They acknowledge its role in the conception of human life, but when procreation is not intended, they advocate other applications for Ching Chi. In the Healing Love practice, this energy is used to heal the internal organs and glands, increase the brain's capacity, and further open the channels of the Microcosmic Orbit. In the more advanced practice of the Sexual Energy Massage, it is also used to replenish and cultivate the blood-producing red marrow of the bones.

We begin this chapter with Penis Power Stretching and Penis Milking, two techniques of Taoist penis enlargement, before detailed instruction in Sexual Energy Massage. Preparation for all of the genital massage techniques given here should include the Hot Hands Warm Up, which should be done before and after every workout of your penis and testicles.

Hot Hands Warm Up

Just as you should warm up your body and muscle tissue before any workout, you should also warm up your penis. This will prepare it for the workout ahead by expanding the tissue and making it more flexible and spongy.

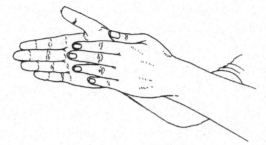

Fig. 2.1. Rub hands.

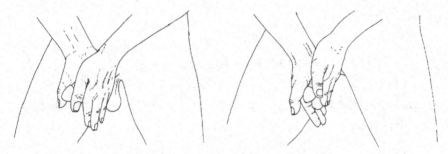

Fig. 2.2. Hold penis and warm up, followed by testicles.

1. Rub your hands warm (fig. 2.1).
2. Hold the penis between the two palms and rub until warm (fig. 2.2).
3. Hold the testicles between the palms and rub them warm.

 ## Penis Power Stretching

To achieve optimal results by stretching your penis, you must understand how the penis works. The penis is made up of cells that enlarge when they fill with blood. These cells are called blood spaces. The blood spaces are within your erectile tissue, also known as the corpora cavernosa. When you stretch the penis, you are stretching all parts of the penis, including the areas that fill with blood. When these areas have stretched to a certain length, the penis will extend longer in both the flaccid and erect state. By naturally exercising blood to fill the spaces, or

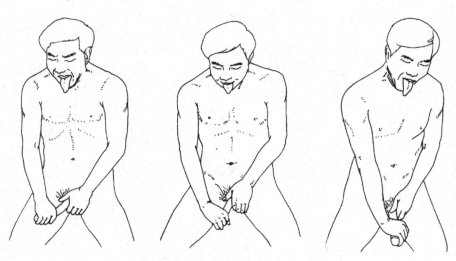

Fig. 2.3. Penis Power Stretching

by stretching the flesh longer, penis enlargement is quite possible with minimal effort.

1. Inhale fully; now exhale and flatten the abdomen while sticking the tongue out (fig. 2.3). Use the thumb and index finger to grip the head of the penis; pull the penis and thrust the tongue out more. Gasp air into the intestines; exhale making the "sh-h-h-h-h-h-h" sound until out of breath.
2. In a standing or sitting position, make sure the penis is in a completely flaccid state and grasp around the head, not so tight as to cause pain but just to ensure a good grip.
3. Pull the penis directly out in front of you until you feel a good stretch in the middle and at the base. Hold this stretch for a 10 count, rest and feel the energy from the sexual organs. Repeat 3 more times.
4. Now slap your penis against the leg about 50 times to get the blood back into where you have been squeezing.
5. Next, grasp around the penis again and exhale, sticking out the tongue. This time, pull to your far left until you feel a good stretch on the right side at the base. Hold this position for a 10 count and repeat. Rest and guide the sexual energy to the crown.

6. Slap the penis against the leg 50 times again.

7. Next, grasp around the penis, sticking out the tongue and holding the breath; this time, pull to your far right until you feel a good stretch on the left side at the base. Hold this position for a 10 count. Repeat 3 more times.

☯ Rotations

1. Grasp around the head of the penis and pull outward until you feel a good stretch.

2. Once extended, begin by rotating the penis in a circular fashion to your left (fig. 2.4). Do not twist it; rather rotate it around in a circular motion. You should feel a good stretch from all areas of the penis and at the base where it connects. Rotate for 30 rotations, rest for a few seconds and gently contract the anus and perineum, guiding the chi up to the crown. Then repeat 3 more times.

3. Slap the penis against your leg 50 times to get the blood flowing again.

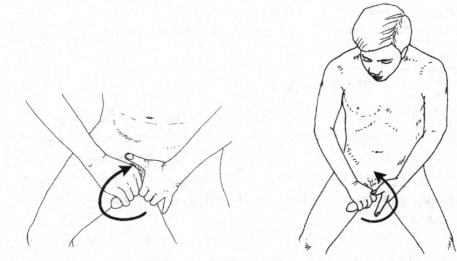

Fig. 2.4. Rotations

4. Do the same rotation technique as before, only this time to your right. Rotate for 30 rotations; rest for a few seconds; then repeat 3 more times.

PENIS MILKING EXERCISES

These exercises stretch out the central tendon-like tissue in your penis, making it longer, both while erect and flaccid. They also promote an increase in testosterone and sperm count. It's very sad that in America alone there are more than thirty million impotent men. A lack of blood circulation to the penis will weaken and shrink the corpora cavernosa and also lessen the sensation and feeling during intercourse, hence promoting impotence. If you have weak erections or have bouts of impotence regularly, this means that you have very poor blood circulation to your penis and testicles. Having proper blood circulation to any part of your body is vital if good health is desired. The milking action in these exercises forces blood into the blood spaces within the corpora cavernosa, not only enlarging the penis but also training the body to accept more blood flow throughout the entire penis. Regular stretching will ensure a healthier and stronger penis after several months of vigorous exercise.

 ## Power Milking

The use of a lubricant while performing this exercise is recommended. Your choice for lubrication is a crucial one; if you choose a lubricant that evaporates easily then you will get tired of reapplying it. Baby oil with Vitamin E is a good lubricant for exercise; it is also nice to apply to the penis and testicles after showering, to keep them healthy and supple.

The tongue is an important part of this exercise because it is connected to all the tendons of the body, especially those of the penis.

When milking, stick the tongue out, and the tongue will get longer as well as the penis. You should always start out by stretching the penis lightly by grasping around the head and pulling outward, while at the same time sticking out the tongue. Rotate your tongue as you rotate your penis in a circular motion. When warming up has been completed, proceed with the milking method.

1. Lightly massage the penis to a partial erection to hold blood within its length.
2. Grasp around the base of the penis shaft with the thumb and forefinger of one hand (see fig. 2.5 on page 48). This retains the blood within the penis. With the other hand grasp all the way around the penis, making an "OK" sign with the forefinger and thumb, and grip tightly.
3. With your thumb and forefinger, squeeze all the way around your penis and slide them forward slowly. This forces the blood within the penis forward into the corpora cavernosa (erectile tissue) and the glans (head).
4. The blood spaces within the penis are forced to expand every time you milk forward. As one hand milks forward to the head, the other hand should be used to grasp around the base of the shaft; once the first hand reaches the head, it should release it and return to the base. Milking should be repeated with alternating hands in this way at a medium to slow pace. Each milking should last 3 to 4 seconds from grasping the base and sliding to the head.

When first starting the milking, some men experience red spots, bumps, or light bruising on the penis head and surrounding areas. Don't worry; this is perfectly normal and will usually subside within the first week of exercise. These effects are simply caused by the stretching of the blood spaces within your penis and the new increased blood circulation.

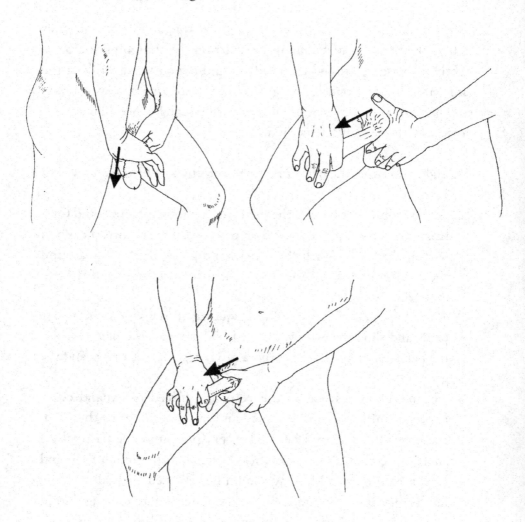

Fig. 2.5. Power Milking

Suggested Timetable

In the beginning, start out by doing 300 milks (5 minutes) a day. Follow this with a 15-minute warm up of rubbing. Do this for one week and be sure to do 100 PC flexes a day in addition. This will aid in the new circulation and strength-building taking place within your penis. The second week will be much harder than the first: 10 minutes of continuous milking followed by 200 PC muscle flexes. Do not ease up unless you happen to feel pain, though this is highly unlikely. Apply a warming up rub for 10 minutes to finish the session.

If the continuous exercise forms painful bruising on the penis, stop all exercising and wait for the bruising to subside. You can always perform PC flexes and stretching.

Milking and Holding

This exercise thickens and lengthens the penis in both its erect and flaccid state. The milk and hold technique is something men should incorporate only after they have already milked for at least 20 minutes to make sure that the penis, and all of the spongy tissue within the penis, is warmed up and stretched out enough that the chance of injury due to overexertion is very minimal.

Warming Up

1. Massage the penis to an erection and flex the PC muscle to make it as hard as possible.
2. Once fully erect, pump the PC 20 times to fully expand the penis as much as possible. Squeeze the PC as hard as possible and hold until the erection reduces somewhat. Now it is time to milk.

Milking

1. Apply lubrication and begin the method of milking.
2. While you milk, visualize the penis lengthening each time you milk down to the head.
3. Milk for 20 minutes continuously without stopping.
4. Once completed, rest for a minute and keep massaging your penis to keep it in a partially erect state. Now you are ready for the milk and hold.

⚙ *Milk and Hold*

1. Begin milking just as you have been, performing each milk with about a 2-second interval.
2. After about 20 milks, milk down a little harder than normal. By doing it firmly the hand should stop when it comes to the head. When this happens, pull hard enough to feel a good stretch in the penis.
3. Repeat the 20-milk set then perform the milk-and-hold with the opposite hand. Continue with this routine over and over again for a total of 500 milkings and 25 milk-and-holds.

⚙ *Cooling Down*

1. At the end of this workout the penis should feel very fatigued and appear quite "pumped" or full looking. Massage the penis to a full, hard erection and flex the PC muscle several times while massaging to enlarge the penis to its fullest potential.
2. Keep massaging and pumping the PC until the urge to ejaculate is quite strong.
3. Once this sensation is reached, flex the PC as hard as possible, cutting off any possibility of semen being able to pass through the ejaculatory duct.
4. Keep flexing until the urge is gone, then repeat. Do this 5 times to cool down.

SEXUAL ENERGY MASSAGE

The Sexual Energy Massage is a beginner's equivalent to Chi Weight Lifting, which requires much more experience. The massage draws sexual energy and hormones into the body and promotes a healthy flow of blood and chi within the sexual center. It also brings more internal energy into the genitals, and increases the production of Ching Chi. Using these techniques, men find that prostate problems can be greatly reduced.

The Sexual Energy Massage often causes enough stimulation to require the Healing Love techniques to avoid sexual arousal. If arousal occurs, draw the activated sexual energy into the Microcosmic Orbit. The Power Lock should be used before the Sexual Energy Massage to prepare for the procedures, and afterward to draw Ching Chi up through the stations of the Microcosmic Orbit. At least two to three sets are recommended at both times.

An extremely important preparation for the Sexual Energy Massage techniques is the Cloth Massage of the sexual center, which stimulates the energy and prepares the sexual organs for the role at hand. The perineum and sacrum are also massaged since they are powerful stimulators of life-force energy.

Cloth Massage

A silk cloth is used to massage the genital area, the perineum, the coccyx, and the sacrum. Silk works well because it develops considerable static energy when rubbed. This is important for the stimulation of chi. First, the silk cloth is applied to activate Ching Chi. The Sexual Energy Massage then releases the Ching Chi to be assimilated into the body. While massaging with the cloth, men should feel their testicles fill with energy as they become firm. Using the cloth should help you feel the chi routes open as they are stimulated.

The Cloth Massage of the sexual center, perineum, and sacrum should also be repeated after the Sexual Energy Massage or Chi Weight Lifting, to replenish the circulation of blood and chi in the sexual center. It is particularly useful in preventing blood coagulation and subsequent blood clots from occurring in the genitals.

1. Hold the cloth using the three middle fingers of either hand. Apply the cloth directly to the genitals in clockwise and counterclockwise motions for 36 rotations in each direction (see fig. 2.6 on page 52).
2. Locate the perineum, and use the cloth to massage it clockwise 36 times, and then counterclockwise 36 times.

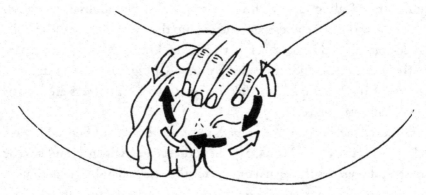

Fig. 2.6. Cloth Massage

3. Apply the cloth to the coccyx and massage its tip, gradually applying more pressure to activate the sacral pump. Massage clockwise and then counterclockwise 36 times. Move up to the sacrum and massage it clockwise, then counterclockwise 36 times (fig. 2.7).

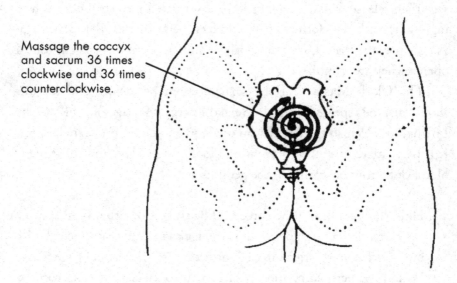

Massage the coccyx
and sacrum 36 times
clockwise and 36 times
counterclockwise.

Fig. 2.7. Massaging the sacrum

Sexual Energy Massage

Sexual Energy Massage includes: Testicle Massage, Duct Elongation Rub, Duct-Stretching Massage, Scrotum and Penis Tendon Stretch, Penis Massage, and Tapping the Testicles.

Testicle Massage

The testicles are very vital and important organs in the body; without them we would be an extinct species. Keeping them in shape will not only give you harder erections, more sex drive, and higher amounts of semen but will also give you a healthier sperm count and chance for conception when you try to have children. The key to proper testicle function and health is better blood circulation to your testicles.

Testicle Massage is a way to consciously connect to the male sexual energy. It is critically important to differentiate these exercises from masturbation. In the Tao, the goal of the practice is to harness this vital energy, not to release it. It is essential that you feel the energy and bring it up into the whole body.

These exercises can be done standing or while sitting on the edge of a chair, without pants. (It is possible to do them with pants on, although they should be very loose, so that the material does not interfere with the massage.) In all of the following exercises, you may wrap the testicles with the cloth as you massage them.

Finger Massage of the Testicles

1. Inhale chi into the testicles as in the Scrotal Compression exercise given in chapter 1. Rub your hands to warm them, and use them to warm the testicles.
2. Hold the right testicle with the right hand. Place the pinky, fourth, third, and second fingertips on the bottom of the testicle. Place the right thumb on the top of the testicle. Hold the left testicle with the left hand in the same manner (see fig. 2.8 on page 54).
3. Use your thumbs to gently press on each testicle, with the other four

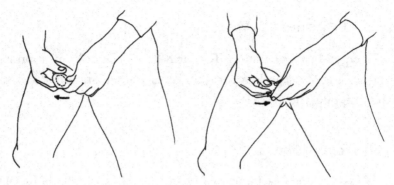

Fig. 2.8. Finger massage of the testicles

fingers holding the bottom of each. Then use your thumbs to massage around the testicles 36 times clockwise and then 36 times counterclockwise (fig. 2.9).

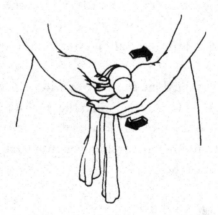

Fig. 2.9. Rub the testicles in each direction up to 36 times.

4. Use your thumbs to hold the testicles in place while the other four fingers of each hand roll them to the left and right or back and forth 36 times in both directions. Draw the energy upward (fig. 2.10).

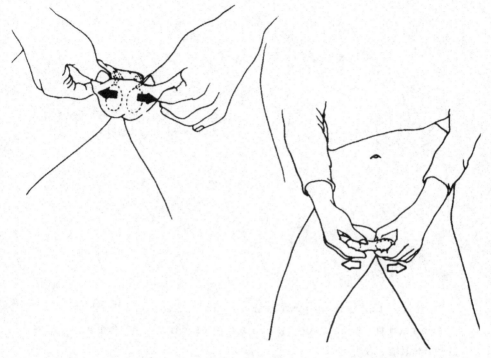

Fig. 2.10. Roll the testicles in each direction up to 36 times.

O Palm Massage of the Testicles

1. Inhale chi into the testicles. Rub your hands together until they are hot, and warm the testicles with them.
2. Move the penis toward the right with the right thumb and forefinger, covering the top of the testicles with the lower edge of the right hand.
3. Place the left palm on the bottom cupping the testicles.
4. Keeping the penis to the right, begin to lightly press the testicles with both hands, and then gently rub the testicles with the left palm 36 times, both clockwise and counterclockwise (see fig. 2.11 on page 56).
5. Warm the hands again, and reverse the hand positions. Then gently rub the testicles with your right palm 36 times in both directions. Draw the energy upward.

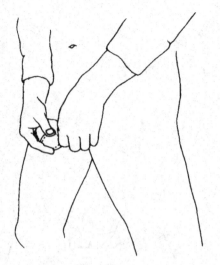

Fig. 2.11. Massage the testicles in the palm of your hand.

◑ Duct Elongation Rub

1. Rub your hands together to warm them, cup the testicles with them, and then trace the ducts extending upward from the rear of the testicles (fig. 2.12).

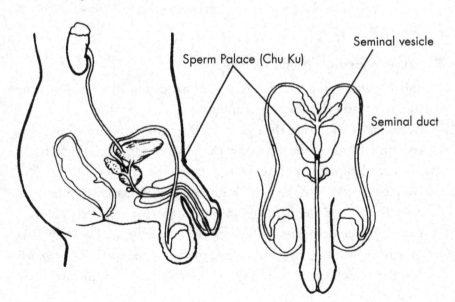

Fig. 2.12. Trace the ducts of the testicles.

2. Gently use your thumbs and index fingers to massage the ducts near the point at which they connect to the testicles. Rub toward the back of each duct with your index finger and use your thumb to rub toward the front. Gradually move along the ducts up toward the body (fig. 2.13). Be careful.

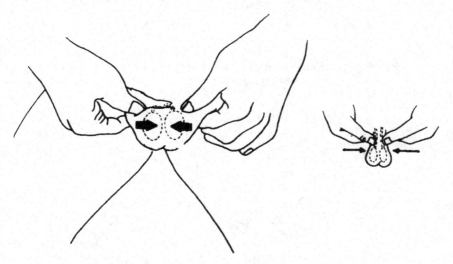

Fig. 2.13. Duct Elongation Rub

3. Reverse finger positions and return downward toward the testicles, now using the thumb to rub the back, and the index fingers to rub the front. Continue rubbing 36 times. Each up and down movement counts as one time. Draw the energy into the Microcosmic Orbit.

Duct-Stretching Massage

1. Use the thumbs and index fingers to hold the ducts, thumbs in front.
2. Use the right thumb to rub toward the left, and use the right index finger to rub and gently pull the right testicle out, stretching the duct.
3. Next use the left thumb to rub toward the right, and the left index finger to rub and gently pull the left testicle out, stretching the duct (see fig. 2.14 on page 58).

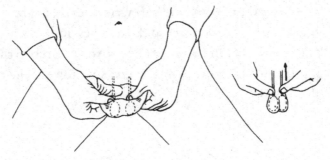

Rub the ducts between thumbs and index fingers,
gently squeezing them upward.

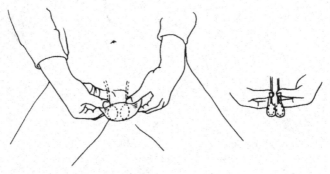

Gently stretch the ducts downward.

Fig. 2.14. Gently stretching the ducts with massage

4. Gently palm massage both testicles, and repeat the stretching.
5. Now you may simultaneously rub the testicles using the thumbs and index fingers of both hands up to 36 times. Draw the energy upward.

After these massaging exercises, your testicles should be stretched out and appear to be hanging lower than normal. They should also appear to be larger. This is due to the increased blood circulated into your testicles from performing the above exercises. You should do these massaging and stretching techniques at least 3–4 times a week, but daily exercise can be performed for absolute optimal testicle health and fertility.

❂ *Scrotum and Penis Tendon Stretch*

1. Warm both hands by rubbing them together.
2. Encircle the base of the penis with the thumb and forefinger as all of the fingers encircle the scrotum, surrounding the testicles (fig. 2.15).

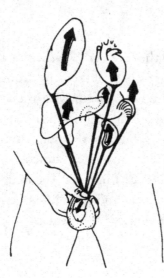

Fig. 2.15. Gently pull down on the penis and testicles as you pull up from the internal organs.

3. Gradually pull the entire groin down toward the tip of the penis as you pull the internal organs up, opposing the outward force with your hand. First, pull straight down with the hand, and then pull down to the left and right in equal counts (fig. 2.16). Simultaneously pull up

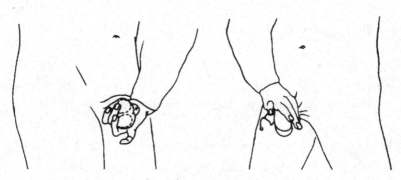

Fig. 2.16. Stretching the scrotum and penis tendons

the internal organs from the perineum. Hold for a while, and then release.

4. Pull downward in a circular motion 9–36 times clockwise and then counterclockwise. Draw the energy upward.

◯ *Penis Massage*

1. Rub the hands together until they are hot. Use the thumbs and index fingers of both hands to hold the base of the penis from the sides.
2. Massage the penis along three lines. Begin with the left line, using the left thumb and index finger to massage from the base of the penis to the tip and back (fig. 2.17). Then use the right thumb and index finger to massage the right line in the same manner.
3. Next place both thumbs and index fingers on the middle line at the base, and massage down to the glans and back. Massage all three lines, counting up and down as one time, up to 36 times.

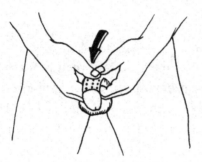

Fig. 2.17. Massage the penis along three lines from the base to the head.

◯ *Tapping the Testicles*

By tapping on the testicles you can directly stimulate the kidney energy of the body. As the kidneys govern sexual energy, tapping the testicles stimulates hormonal production through the entire endocrine system.

1. Stand in a wide stance or sit on the edge of a chair. Rub your palms together until warm, then use the left hand to grasp the penis and pull it upward.

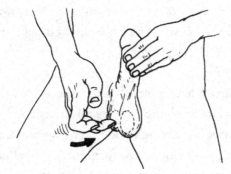

Fig. 2.18. Tap the testicles lightly.

2. Inhale chi directly into the testicles, slightly pulling them up, and hold your breath. Clench the teeth, contract the perineum and anus, but only contract the testicles very slightly.

3. Use the fingertips of the right hand to lightly tap the right testicle (fig 2.18). Do not tap so hard that it is painful, but tap hard enough to feel it all over the lower abdomen. Tap in sets of 6, 7, or 9. Exhale, rest, and draw the energy up the spine. Use the same procedures with the left testicle.

☯ Resting

Resting after massaging is very important. Use your mind to channel your breathing into long, smooth, soft breaths. Then draw the energy of these breaths to the point on which you are working.

Suggested Timetable

Practice the Sexual Energy Massage lightly for the first ten days. If you do not have time for all the techniques, try at least one of them daily. You can divide the exercises so that different sets are practiced on alternate days. Practice in sets of up to 36 repetitions, as long as you are comfortable with this regimen. Forego practice, or at least decrease it, whenever you do not feel comfortable. Once you are skilled, these exercises can be completed very quickly.

After ten days you may increase the force of each exercise as you decrease the number of repetitions per set. You may also use fewer sets per exercise. After fifty days, further increase the force as you decrease the repetitions and sets, spending more time on the palm and finger massages. After this, those who have taken instruction in Bone Marrow Nei Kung may feel ready to begin Chi Weight Lifting.

Warning: If you know that you have a blood clot in the area of the scrotum, consult a physician before applying the Sexual Energy Massage or Chi Weight Lifting techniques. Although the massage techniques presented here help to prevent blood clots from forming, medical advice is necessary to determine their safety with existing blood clots.

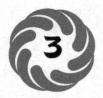

Chi Weight Lifting

Chi Weight Lifting is included in this text solely for the documentation of its procedure to serve as a guide for instructors and trained students of the Universal Healing Tao. It is not intended for beginning students. Universal Healing Tao cannot and will not be held responsible for any reader of this book who attempts Chi Weight Lifting without first receiving qualified instruction.

The ancient Taoist masters discovered that the genitals were connected to the organs and glands in an area of the perineum called the Chi Muscle, which encompasses the anal, perineal, and pubococcygeus muscles (see fig. 3.1 on page 64). With this knowledge they developed the Healing Love techniques, using the Chi Muscle to create an upward flow of sexual energy into the higher centers of the body. They eventually learned to increase this chi flow by developing the fascia, the connective tissue around the organs and glands. In the Chi Weight Lifting practice the fascia is engaged by the organs and glands to lift weights externally anchored to the genitals. The beneficial aspects of strengthening the internal system through the fascia became an integral part of Bone Marrow Nei Kung.

Originally men accomplished Chi Weight Lifting by placing stones in a basket and hanging the basket from their groins. Today, light weights are used to draw a special formula of sexual energy from the genitals upward into the body. This sexual energy, or Ching Chi, is combined with external energy and compressed into the skeletal structure. As sexual energy transforms into

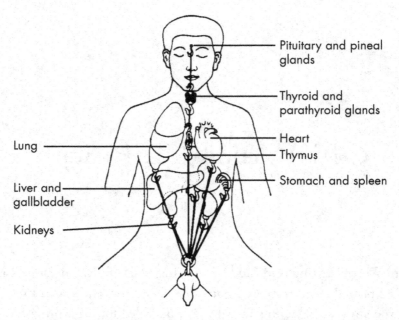

Pituitary and pineal glands

Thyroid and parathyroid glands

Lung

Heart

Thymus

Liver and gallbladder

Stomach and spleen

Kidneys

Fig. 3.1. Sexual organs are joined to all of the organs, glands, tendons, and muscles.

life-force energy, Chi Weight Lifting enhances the life-force of those who practice it. The genitals are replenished by the rejuvenated organs and glands as the transformed energy returns through the Microcosmic Orbit.

In addition to Sexual Energy Massage and Chi Weight Lifting, Bone Marrow Nei Kung also includes the practices of Bone Breathing, Bone Compression, and Hitting with a bundle of wire rods or rattan sticks. Bone Breathing uses the power of the mind, along with deep, relaxed inhalations, to establish an inward flow of external energy through the fingertips and toes. This energy is used to complement previously stored sexual energy, which is released into the body through the Sexual Energy Massage or Chi Weight Lifting and then compressed into the bones using Bone Compression. The Hitting techniques are employed to detoxify the body, stimulate the lymphatic and nervous systems, and compress chi into the bones. A summary of the Bone Breathing and Bone Compression techniques is provided in chapter 5 of this book, while detailed instruction in Hitting can be found in chapter 4 of *Bone Marrow Nei Kung* (Destiny Books, 2006).

BENEFITS OF
CHI WEIGHT LIFTING

In Chi Weight Lifting, an upward counterforce is created by the internal organs and glands to resist weight that is placed upon the genitals.

Strengthens the Fascial Network

The upward counterforce created by the organs is strengthened by the chi released from the sexual center as the internal system engages the fascia to pull up against the weight. The fascia, therefore, contributes greatly to the distribution of energy. It also serves as the connection between the genitalia and the pelvic and urogenital diaphragms. When this connection is loose, the Chi Muscle and the diaphragms allow the organs to drop their weight onto the perineum, thereby reducing the chi pressure. When the connection is kept strong, the organs and glands are held in place and the chi pressure is maintained.

Creates Powerful Urogenital
and Pelvic Diaphragms

The human body has many diaphragms holding the internal organs and glands in place, such as the thoracic, pelvic, and urogenital diaphragms. During Chi Weight Lifting these contribute greatly to the upward counterforce deployed against the downward pull of the weights anchored to the genitals (see fig. 3.2 on page 66). The pelvic and urogenital diaphragms, considered the floor of the organs, and the Chi Muscle are all strengthened by this practice, which helps to prevent any loss of energy through them. Their increased strength also helps to alleviate the protruding abdomen caused by organs stacking up on the pelvic area (see fig. 3.3 on page 66).

Chi Weight Lifting is credited with many other benefits related to the improved functioning of the diaphragms, such as the lifting of dropped kidneys. Furthermore, the practice helps to seal the openings of the anus and sex organ to prevent the leakage of chi. Taoists believe that this helps to redirect the spirit away from these openings as one prepares to finally

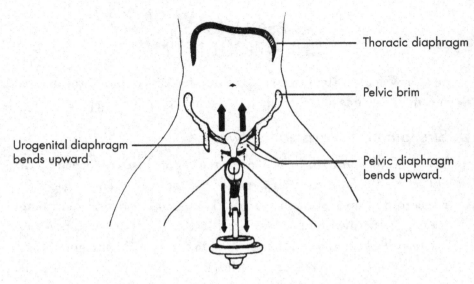

Thoracic diaphragm

Pelvic brim

Urogenital diaphragm
bends upward.

Pelvic diaphragm
bends upward.

Fig. 3.2. The pelvic and urogenital diaphragms
provide counterforce to the weights.

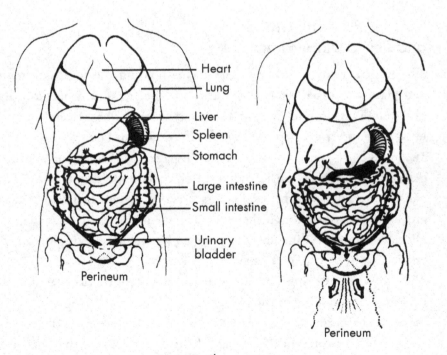

Heart
Lung
Liver
Spleen
Stomach
Large intestine
Small intestine
Urinary
bladder
Perineum

Perineum

Fig. 3.3. The organs

leave the body. The upward flow of energy that is developed through Taoist practices will point toward the crown as the proper exit for the spirit to use at the end of life.

Delays the Aging Process

The release of sexual hormones stimulates the pituitary gland to prevent the production of an aging hormone. It has been proposed that one function of this gland may be to measure the growth of mutated reproductive cells. Scientific studies have found some evidence that the aging hormone is released when these mutations are allowed to increase beyond a certain level. Theoretically their growth should be impeded by a healthy reserve of sexual hormones. Otherwise, upon sensing the reduced presence of Ching Chi within the body, the pituitary gland can cause a premature death by producing the aging hormone. It is therefore wise to maintain sexual energy and hormones through the Taoist practices.

Stimulates the Brain

The right side of the brain is also influenced by the sexual hormones to promote the healing and rejuvenation of the body. Since Ching Chi revitalizes the internal system and regenerates the bone marrow, hormonal stimulation of the brain greatly enhances these processes. This effect also serves Taoist spiritual work because practitioners find it to be an invigorating experience on all levels. The health of the body and the mind directly affects the spirit.

EQUIPMENT AND EXTERNAL PREPARATIONS

Cloth for Lifting the Weight

The same silk cloth used for the Sexual Energy Massage is then used to lift the weight with a special holding apparatus. Two sizes of cloth can be used to lift the weight, depending on the method chosen for practice. The smaller cloth, which is used for lifting the weight from a table or chair, should measure approximately 3½ by 8 inches. If you choose to lift the weight from the floor, the length of the cloth can vary according to the length of your legs. When the cloth has been cut to size, you can sew the edges to prevent unraveling and to avoid abrasions of the skin.

Equipment

A special device is required to hold the weights (fig. 3.4). To make this device, a 10-inch length of 1-inch diameter galvanized pipe is needed for an apparatus to be used from the floor. An 8-inch length of pipe is needed for an apparatus to be used from a chair. (Either size is adaptable to either method if necessary.) A ¼-inch hole should be drilled through the pipe ½ inch from either end.

Secure a piece of chain two links long to the pipe with a ¼-inch bolt inserted through the hole and fastened by a nut and washer at its end. At the end of the chain, a heavy ring 1½ inches in diameter is attached. Any of several different types of clamps (used in standard barbell sets) may be used on the opposite end of the pipe to hold the weights. After the silk cloth has been tied gently, but firmly, around the groin, it can then be attached to the ring in order to lift the entire weight-holding apparatus.

Some men can begin Chi Weight Lifting with a 2½-pound weight. It is safer, however, to start with the apparatus alone, or with one or two weight clamps attached to it. The weight of two clamps should equal 1 pound, plus the weight of the apparatus itself. Add on more weight gradually, but only as much as you feel comfortable with. Do not advance to heavier weights unless you can lift the current weight easily for one minute.

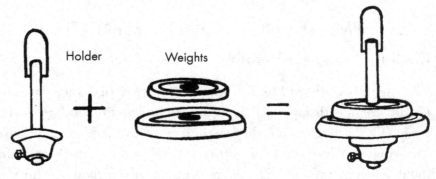

Fig. 3.4. Weight-lifting device

External Preparations

The room in which you practice should be quiet and well ventilated, but not cold. Keep a hard chair available for your meditation and as a place to rest the weight, unless you lift from the floor. The best time for these exercises is in the morning after you shower and relieve your bladder and bowels. If you can, face the sun as you practice in the early morning hours, but never look directly into it at any time.

The optimum condition for Chi Weight Lifting is when the testicles are slightly loose, but firm. If the testicles are too tight and close to the body, none of the tying methods will work. Massage the testicles until they loosen. If the scrotum is very loose and hanging weakly and the testicles feel weak, it is not safe to practice weight lifting. Practice only the massage techniques.

The strength of the testicles can be felt internally rather than with the fingers. In other words, when they are massaged, their resilience and ability to withstand the massage without pain will indicate their condition. A slight pain from the first massage may be the result of a beginner's apprehensions. Do not begin to practice weight lifting until you are comfortable emotionally as well as physically.

Weight-Lifting Goals

The Universal Tao does not recommend that anyone try to lift more than 10 pounds without supervision. On the basis of this book, 10 pounds should be considered the absolute maximum goal. It is certainly no shame to lift less than the 1 or 2 pounds recommended for beginners. If you choose to lift beyond 5 pounds, exercise more than the usual caution.

Warning: Lifting heaver weights without supervision is both foolish and contrary to the recommendations of this book. In systems where excessive weights are used for practice, broken veins or blood clots have occurred in some overzealous men, resulting in serious injury. (There are no statistics available concerning possible deaths that may have occurred.) Contact the Universal Tao Center for information on instruction.

PREPARATORY EXERCISES
FOR CHI WEIGHT LIFTING

Chi Weight Lifting should be preceded and followed by both the Power Lock given in chapter 1 and the Sexual Energy Massage techniques given in chapter 2. Although not all six techniques are required, the Sexual Energy Massage must be repeated after the weights are removed to restore the circulation of blood and chi to the sexual center. This ensures that the genital area will be clear of any blood coagulation that can lead to blood clots.

Two additional practices should also precede Chi Weight Lifting: the Increasing Chi Pressure and Increasing Kidney Pressure exercises.

 ## Increasing Chi Pressure

This exercise is done before the Power Lock exercise in order to ensure that the abdomen is full of chi.

1. Place the middle finger of each hand about 1½ inches below the navel (fig. 3.5).
2. Concentrate on the lower tan tien as you inhale chi into it, expanding the point with the resulting pressure. Your mental power will increase the energy flow to this area.

Increasing Kidney Pressure

1. Stand in a Horse stance with your feet slightly wider than shoulder width.
2. Rub your hands together until they are warm, and then apply their warmth to the kidneys by placing your energized palms on them from the back (fig. 3.6).
3. Bend your upper body forward slightly as you inhale, and pull up the left and right sides of the anus as you draw chi up to the kidneys.
4. Exhale, and deflate the kidneys.
5. Follow this sequence up to 36 times, and finish by warming the hands and again placing them on the kidneys.

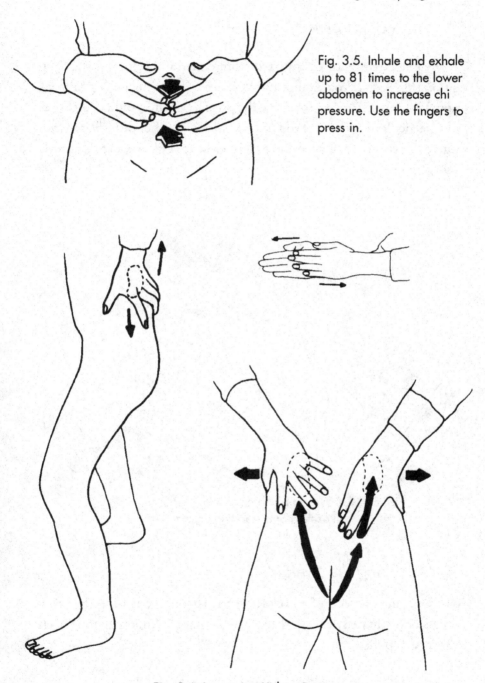

Fig. 3.5. Inhale and exhale up to 81 times to the lower abdomen to increase chi pressure. Use the fingers to press in.

Fig. 3.6. Increasing Kidney Pressure

Chi Weight Lifting

Chi Weight Lifting can be initiated from either a kneeling or standing position (fig. 3.7). If you cannot kneel, set the weight on a chair in front of you. It may be necessary to relieve the pressure of the weights quickly at times, particularly if they are too heavy and the knot beneath the testicles is tight. For this reason, keep the weight close to a place where it can be quickly removed.

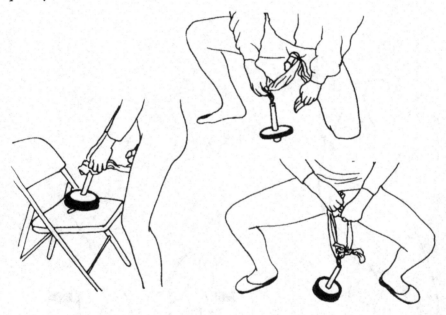

Fig. 3.7. Chi Weight Lifting can be initiated from either a kneeling or a standing position.

Attaching the Weight

Consider tying one end of the cloth to the ring while leaving the other end in a loop—folded beneath the knot—so that the knot will undo itself if that end is pulled.

Warning: Do not tie the cloth around the testicles alone.

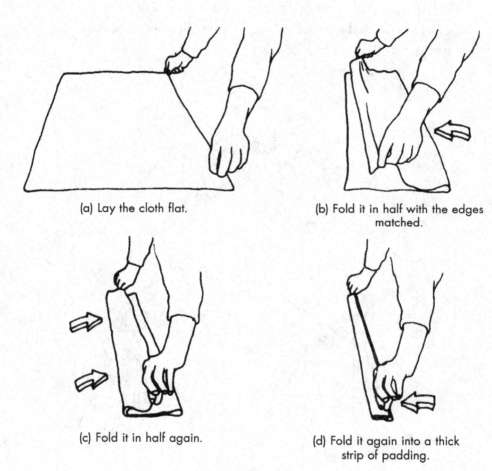

(a) Lay the cloth flat.

(b) Fold it in half with the edges matched.

(c) Fold it in half again.

(d) Fold it again into a thick strip of padding.

Fig. 3.8. Folding the cloth

1. Fold the cloth lengthwise several times to a width of about one inch (fig. 3.8). This creates a thick padding.
2. Hold the cloth beneath the perineum, and bring it up behind the testicles. Be sure that the edge of the cloth is folded away from the skin so that it does not cut into the groin.
3. Wrap both ends of the cloth upward around the penis and testicles, and secure the cloth at the surface of the penis base by tying a knot.

Note: If you prefer, you can place the cloth on top of the penis and tie the knot beneath the testicles. In either case, the knot must eventually be positioned at the perineum (fig. 3.9).

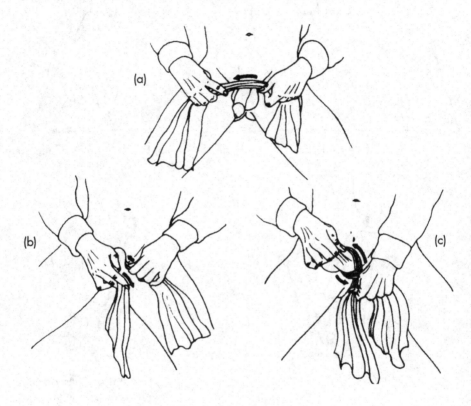

Fig. 3.9. Tying the silk cloth around the genitals

4. Move the knot behind the testicles and beneath the perineum. The ends of cloth should hang to the floor. Before tightening the knot, you can use one end to create a loop between the knot and the groin so that the cloth and apparatus can be quickly removed.

5. Contract the muscles of the perineum region and tighten the knot. The penis and testicles should bulge slightly from the pressure to insure against slippage. Do not cut off the circulation to the testicles.

6. Tie one end of the cloth to the weight that you have placed on the floor or on a chair. If the weight is on the floor, tie the cloth to it from a kneeling position.
7. To remove the weight at the end of practice, kneel in front of the chair—or near the floor—and untie the cloth attached to the holding apparatus, then remove the cloth from the groin.

⟳ Testing and Lifting the Weight

1. Slowly stand up, holding the cloth or the weight in your hand, and assume a weight-lifting stance, with the feet parallel at about shoulder width, and the knees slightly bent. Use your index and middle fingers to test the weight and determine whether or not it is too heavy.
2. Inhale a sip of air and pull up the anus, perineum, and genitals. Inhale again, and pull up both sides of the anus as you draw chi into the left and right kidneys respectively.
3. Press the tongue firmly up to the roof of your mouth to increase your internal power. Increasing pressure on this connection will accelerate the upward force of the chi.
4. Then, slowly release the cloth or the string from your fingers until you are sustaining the weight from the sexual organ. With the fingers of one hand nearby, feel the pull of the weight, and determine whether or not your genitals can sustain it. Be certain that you are reasonably comfortable.
5. Begin to pull against the weight using internal strength, particularly from the kidneys.
6. Inhale, pull up the right, left, front, and back sides of the anus and wrap the energy around the kidneys (see fig. 3.10 on page 76).
7. Gently swing the weight, drawing the energy up to the coccyx and then to the sacrum. You can practice up to the sacrum for the first few weeks. When you feel more energy you can gradually move it up the spine to T11, C7, the Jade Pillow, and all the way to the crown. When you are

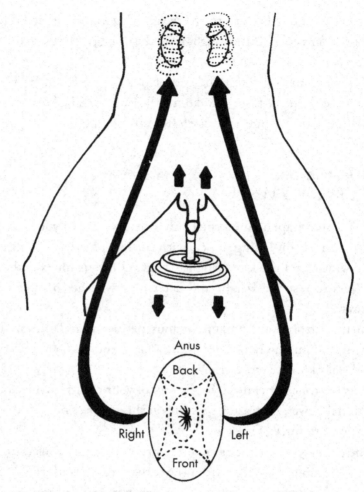

Fig. 3.10. When you feel the pull of the weight, inhale and pull up the right, left, front, and back parts of the anus. Wrap the chi around the kidneys.

ready to store the energy, press your tongue to your palate and bring the energy down to the navel, completing the Microcosmic Orbit.

In advanced practice, a separate round is used to lift the same weight from the internal organs and glands. Rather than remove the weight you may hold it as you rest between rounds.

8. To finish the practice, kneel as you place the weight on the chair or the floor again, and remove the weight-holding apparatus. Untie the

cloth after the apparatus has been removed. The Power Lock should be practiced immediately afterward.

◉ Swinging the Weight

Swinging the weight gives the practitioner control over the amount of pressure on the groin, which is why lighter weights are recommended. The chi from the fascial connection between the perineum and the kidneys is used to pull the weight. In the beginning swing the weights gently as you determine the amount of pressure that is comfortable for you.

1. Inhale as you contract the anus and perineum. Swing the attached weight from 36 to 49 times (fig. 3.11). Synchronize your breathing with each swing. Inhale as the weight swings forward, and exhale as it swings backward. Pull up against the weight internally with each forward swing, and draw the energy up to the coccyx, the sacrum, and then all the way through the Microcosmic Orbit. Each completed swing back and forth should approximate 1 second.

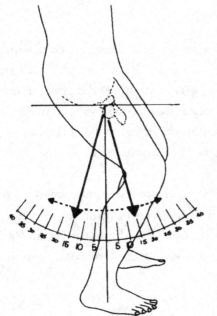

Fig. 3.11. Swing the weight at an angle between 15 and 30 degrees.

2. After a week, try to swing the weight for 60 counts. More pressure results from the counterforce exerted by the Chi Muscle when heavier weights are swung, but rather than progressing rapidly to heavier weights, it is wiser to increase the pressure with lighter weights by adding more power to each swing. The lighter weights should be used to their maximum potential, thereby strengthening the Chi Muscle and producing more hormones.

⚙ Finish with the Power Lock and Massage Techniques

Practice the Power Lock for at least two or three rounds after releasing the weight. Then apply the Cloth Massage and the Sexual Energy Massage techniques. Rest, and practice the Microcosmic Orbit meditation to circulate the tremendous energy you have generated, finally collecting it in the navel.

⚙ Lifting Weights from the Microcosmic Orbit

After you have practiced for 2 to 4 weeks, and feel comfortable with Chi Weight Lifting, begin to lift the weight from the stations of the Microcosmic Orbit. As you bring the chi up into the sacrum and higher centers, use this energy to pull the weight from each station. Take your time, and don't rush. Each point may require 1 or 2 weeks before you feel the flow of the Microcosmic Orbit working as part of the counterforce.

1. Sacrum: When you lift the weights from the sexual organs, pull up the front, back, right, and left of the anus to bring the energy up to the sacrum (fig. 3.12). Hold it there. Breathe normally, and gently swing the weights. Feel a line of energy from the sexual center up to the sacrum.

2. Door of Life: Once you feel the chi in the sacrum, bring it to the Door of Life on the spine, opposite the navel (fig. 3.13). Hold the chi

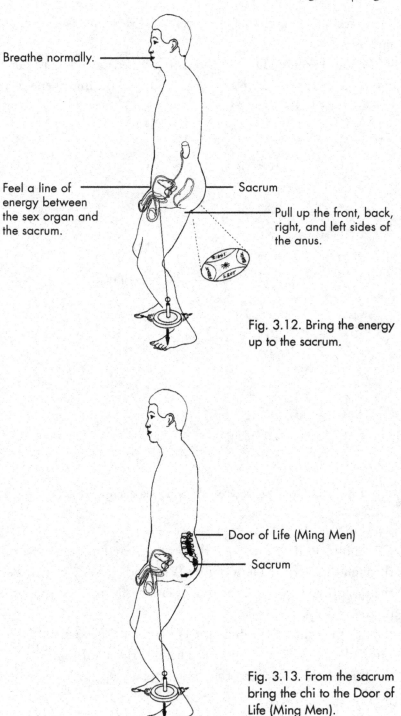

Breathe normally.

Feel a line of
energy between
the sex organ and
the sacrum.

Sacrum

Pull up the front, back,
right, and left sides of
the anus.

Fig. 3.12. Bring the energy
up to the sacrum.

Door of Life (Ming Men)

Sacrum

Fig. 3.13. From the sacrum
bring the chi to the Door of
Life (Ming Men).

there, and continue to swing the weights. Every time you swing, pull up more.

3. T11 point: From the Door of Life, bring the energy up to T11 on the spine, opposite the solar plexus (fig. 3.14). Feel the line of energy as it moves up to T11.

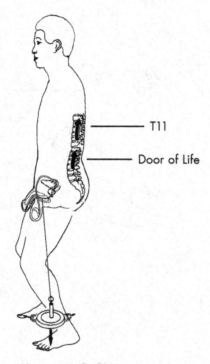

T11

Door of Life

Fig. 3.14. From the Door of Life bring the energy up to T11.

4. C7 point: Pull the energy from the sexual center, passing it through the sacrum, Door of Life, T11, and up to C7 at the base of the neck (fig. 3.15). Feel the line of energy from the sexual organs up to C7.

5. Base of the skull: Next draw the chi through the sacrum, Door of Life, T11, and C7, and up to the base of the skull (fig. 3.16). Feel the line of chi flow from the sexual organs up to the base of the skull.

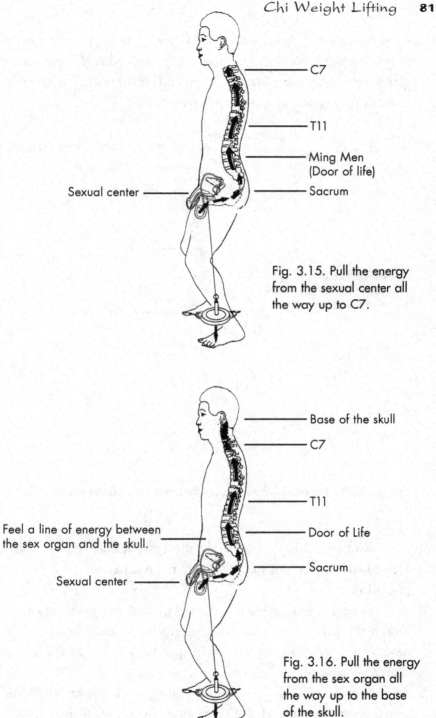

C7

T11

Ming Men
(Door of life)

Sexual center

Sacrum

Fig. 3.15. Pull the energy
from the sexual center all
the way up to C7.

Base of the skull

C7

T11

Feel a line of energy between
the sex organ and the skull.

Door of Life

Sacrum

Sexual center

Fig. 3.16. Pull the energy
from the sex organ all
the way up to the base
of the skull.

6. Crown point and the pineal gland: Draw the chi up to the Crown point where the pineal gland is (fig. 3.17). Remember that the sexual glands are closely related to the pineal and pituitary glands. You may feel this connection as these glands are stimulated.

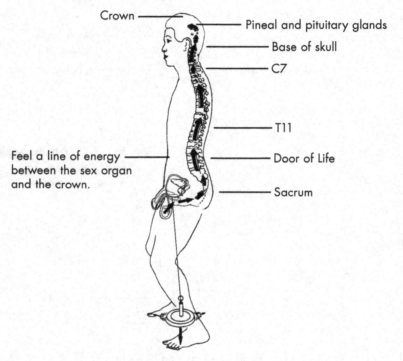

Fig. 3.17. Pull the energy from the sex organ all the way to the crown.

7. The "third eye": Bring the chi to the third eye, or mid-eyebrow point, also called the "Crystal Room," where the pituitary gland is located (fig. 3.18).

8. With the tongue on the palate, bring the chi down to the throat center, the heart center, the solar plexus, and finally down to the navel (fig. 3.19). The overflow will spill back down to the sexual center.

9. At this point you have successfully brought the energy from the sexual organs up through the spine, over the top of the head, down

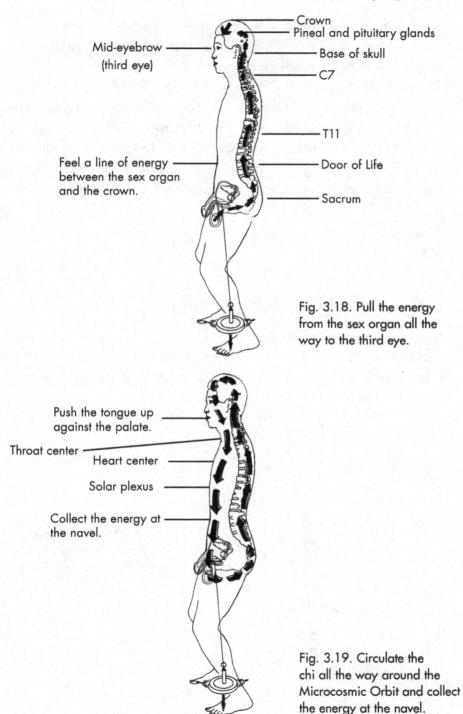

Crown
Pineal and pituitary glands
Mid-eyebrow
(third eye)
Base of skull
C7

T11

Feel a line of energy
between the sex organ
and the crown.
Door of Life

Sacrum

Fig. 3.18. Pull the energy
from the sex organ all the
way to the third eye.

Push the tongue up
against the palate.

Throat center
Heart center

Solar plexus

Collect the energy at
the navel.

Fig. 3.19. Circulate the
chi all the way around the
Microcosmic Orbit and collect
the energy at the navel.

the front to the navel, and back again to the sexual organs, circulating it through the Microcosmic Orbit. This process refines and enhances chi as it moves through the energy centers.

10. Once the Microcosmic Orbit is open to the flowing sexual energy, all you need do is pull the energy up to the head, and then down to the navel through the tongue. Concentrate on drawing the energy up, circulating it in the Microcosmic Orbit, and storing it in the navel. The chi will flow very quickly through all the centers. You will no longer need to bring it up through the points of the spine one by one.

Advanced Chi Weight Lifting Using the Internal Organs

Kidneys Help Pull the Weight

In the beginning stages of Chi Weight Lifting, it is the power of the kidneys that provides real internal counterforce (fig. 3.20). Once you can feel that power, it becomes easier to tap the force of the other organs to help

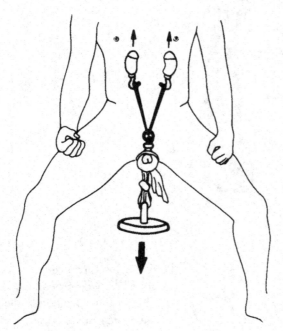

Fig. 3.20. In the beginning stages of Chi Weight Lifting it is the kidneys that provide the internal counterforce.

lift heavier weights. As you begin to increase the weight, start to use the strength of the other organs and glands to increase the upward counterforce. The main secret of internal power is to press the tongue against the roof of the mouth as you direct the force of the organ's energy toward it.

1. Always begin by pulling the energy up to the head several times to make sure of its flow within the Microcosmic Orbit.
2. Inhale with small sips, pull up the left side of the anus, and spiral the energy to the left kidney. Inhale again, pull up the right side of the anus, and spiral the energy into the right kidney (fig. 3.21). Hold the energy there, and feel the chi in the kidneys pull up toward the tongue, resisting the weight. Some people report that they can immediately feel the kidneys as they help lift the weight.

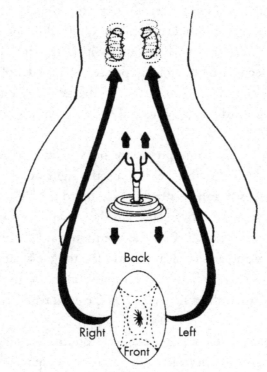

Back

Right   Left

Front

Fig. 3.21. When you feel the weight, inhale and pull up the right and left side of the anus. Wrap the energy around the kidneys.

3. Exhale, maintaining the pulling action of the perineum and kidneys, and then breathe normally. With each swing, pull up more on the sexual organs and kidneys. Practice from 36 to 49 swings.

◉ *Spleen and Liver Pull the Weight*

Always keep the chest relaxed during these procedures. You can practice lifting from the spleen and liver as separate exercises or together as one exercise.

1. Spleen: Start again on the left side by pulling up the left side of the anus and perineum. Become aware of the spleen situated beneath the left side of the rib cage (fig. 3.22). (The spleen is located toward the back, slightly above the left kidney and adrenal gland.) Contract the left anus as you inhale a small sip of air. Pull the chi up to the spleen and left kidney with one more sip. Wrap the chi around and into the spleen. Keep the tongue pressed to the roof of your mouth. Then, as you feel its connection to the genitals, pull the spleen energy up toward the tongue, and lift the genitals, thereby lifting the weight.

2. Liver: Practice the same procedure on the liver, which lies under the right side of the rib cage. Pull up the right side of the anus and perineum. As you inhale, draw the chi up to the right kidney. Then become aware of your liver, and pull the chi up to it twice. Pack and wrap the liver with chi. Pull the energy toward the back, near the right kidney and adrenal gland. Push the tongue against the roof of your mouth. Then, as you feel its connection to the genitals, draw the liver energy up to the tongue. Pull up the genitals, thereby lifting the weight.

3. Combine the procedures of the spleen from the left side and the liver from the right side in order to help lift the weight. Pull their combined energies up toward the tongue.

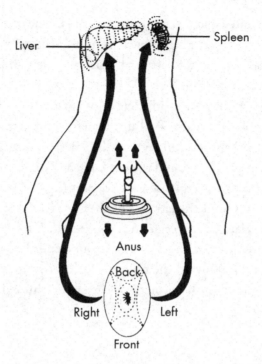

Fig. 3.22. Inhale and pull up the left side of the anus, directing the energy to the spleen. Inhale and pull up the right side of the anus, directing the energy to the liver. Wrap the energy around these organs.

☸ Lifting with the Lungs

Lifting a weight with the lungs is an advanced procedure and is more difficult than lifting with other organs and glands. Before you try to apply Chi Weight Lifting using the lungs, practice pulling energy up to each of the lower organs in succession, drawing the organ energy up toward the tongue. Pull up the chi of the lower organs until you actually feel each lung contracting. Only lift with the lungs when you feel the energy reach them from the lower organs. Don't use force in this exercise. Use your chi to lift the weight in conjunction with light muscular action and strong mental power.

Each step should first be practiced separately. Later, all of the steps can be combined into one practice. The procedure is as follows.

1. First inhale and expand the upper left stomach near the left rib cage. Inhale again, and pull the stomach in toward the spine, up to the left rib cage, and then to the left lung. Push your left shoulder and side slightly toward the front.

2. Inhale a sip of air, pull up the left anus toward the left lung as you pull up the sexual organs. Pull up the left kidney, and then pull up the spleen. Feel the left kidney and the spleen assisting the left lung. Contract the muscles around the left lung, and draw the chi up to and around that lung through the lower organs (fig. 3.23).

3. Pull the chi up from the left side of the anus to the bladder, left kidney, adrenal gland, and spleen until you feel the lung contracting. Feel all of these organs in a line between the lung and the genitals. Use the organs to pull up toward the tongue. Push your tongue hard against the roof of your mouth as you draw the chi up through the organs to the left lung.

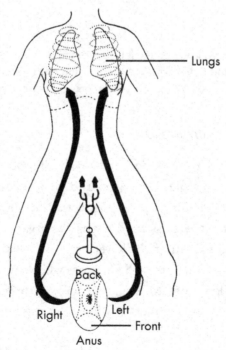

Fig. 3.23. Inhale and pull up both sides of the anus, directing the energy through the lower organs to the lungs. Wrap the energy around the lungs.

4. Use the same procedure with the right side until a line can be felt passing through the associated organs, such as the right kidney and liver, to your right lung. When you feel the fascial connection to the genitals, use all of the lower organs to pull the genitals up toward the lungs, helping them lift the weights. Once you can exert this power from the lungs, you may eliminate the procedure of expanding the stomach area.

☯ Lifting with the Heart (Cautiously!)

As you progress to the heart, be sure that you are in control of the other organs first. The heart and lungs can easily become congested with energy, which can cause chest pain and difficult breathing. If you have this problem, tap the area around the heart and practice the Healing Sound associated with that organ. (The Six Healing Sounds are described in chapter 5 of this book and in *The Six Healing Sounds*, Destiny Books, 2009.)

Before lifting the weight, practice drawing up the chi and wrapping it into and around the heart. Proceed as follows with caution:

1. Create a ball of energy in the center of the abdomen, above the navel (see fig. 3.24 on page 90).
2. Inhale a sip of air, pull up the front part of the anus, and expand the chi ball upward toward the rib cage.
3. Inhale another sip, draw the chi ball inward, and then pull it up under the sternum. Expand it under the sternum toward the back and to the left side.
4. Push your tongue up against the roof of your mouth, push the left shoulder toward the front, and feel your heart.
5. Slowly exhale, and regulate your breath.
6. When you are well practiced, eliminate the step of expanding the abdominal area. Simply inhale in sips, pull up the front part of the anus as you pull up the sexual organs. Pull up the abdomen to the rib cage, and pull the chi to the heart, using the power of the heart. Wrap the chi into and around the heart.

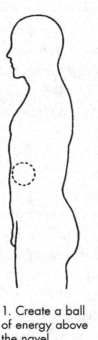

1. Create a ball of energy above the navel.

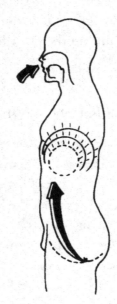

2. Inhale and pull up the front part of the anus, and expand the "chi ball" beneath the sternum.

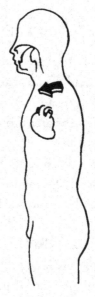

3. Press the tongue against the roof of the mouth and push the left shoulder forward. Feel the heart.

Fig. 3.24. Expanding a chi ball beneath the sternum

7. Pull up the genitals, bladder, kidneys, liver, and spleen toward the tongue. Contract the muscles around the heart and lungs, and successively pull the chi up through each of the lower organs. Start lifting with the lower organs, and draw the chi upward through each of them to reach the heart.

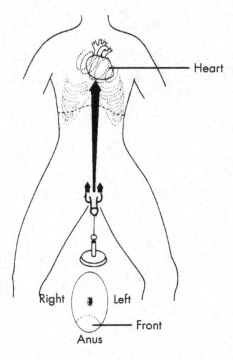

Heart

Right Left

Front

Anus

Fig. 3.25. Pull up the front part of the anus and direct the energy to the heart.
Wrap the energy around the heart.

8. When you are ready to practice Chi Weight Lifting from the heart,
simply pull up the front part of the anus, the genitals, bladder,
kidneys, liver, and spleen to the heart (fig. 3.25). Employ the power of
the heart and lungs to help the other organs and glands pull against
the genitals, thereby lifting the weight.

Thymus Gland Adds Power to the Heart and Lungs

Contracting the muscles around the thymus, heart, and lungs will greatly
increase their combined force.

1. First sink the sternum to the back and push the lungs toward the
thymus under the sternum as you exhale.

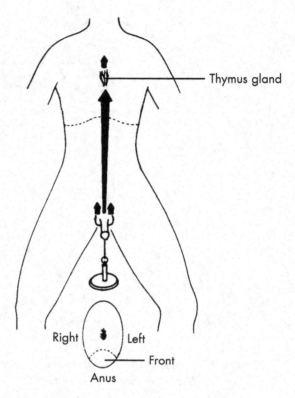

Fig. 3.26. Pull up the weight by contracting the thymus.

2. Then connect the chi of the heart to the thymus, which is in close proximity to the heart. This will enable them to work together to draw chi up through the lower organs, pull up the genitals, and lift the weight (fig. 3.26).

Pulling from the Pituitary and Pineal Glands

The tongue and eyes act as major tools in exerting control over the pituitary and pineal glands.

1. Practice this by first pressing the tongue to the palate and turning the eyes upward. Then contract the eye muscles toward the middle of the brain and the pituitary gland.

2. Contract the cranium from all sides: Squeeze in from the crown, the base of the lower jaw near the throat, and the front, back, left, and right sides of the skull, gently compressing the center of the brain. Concentrating on the center point behind the mid-eyebrow, prepare to draw the energy up to the pituitary gland. You are using the muscles of the skull to increase the pressure on this area.

3. Contract the middle part of the anus, and pull the chi all the way up into the brain.

4. Contract the lungs, heart, and thymus gland, and push their energy up toward the center of the brain. The pituitary gland pulls energy from the thymus gland, heart, lungs, spleen, liver, adrenal glands, kidneys, bladder, and sexual organs. All of these parts will then work together to pull up the weight (fig. 3.27).

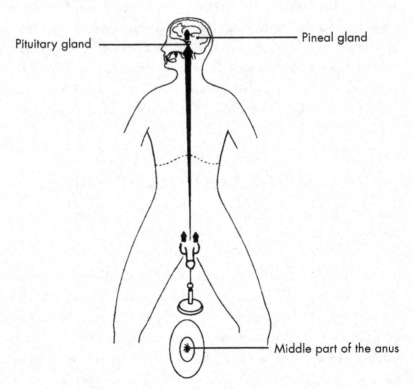

Fig. 3.27. Contract the middle part of the anus and pull up all the way to the brain. Lift the weight by contracting the pituitary gland.

5. Repeat the practice, now focusing on the pineal gland at the crown of the head.

○ Circulate Energy through the Microcosmic Orbit

Since all the steps of this exercise are extremely powerful, use caution. After you have finished all of the steps mentioned above, circulate the energy in the Microcosmic Orbit several times, collecting it in the navel. This is a very important safety measure. Finally, remove the weight.

○ After Chi Weight Lifting

After you have released the weights, practice the Power Lock 2 or 3 times up to the crown, and massage the sexual organs again. First massage the genitals, sacrum, and perineum with the cloth, then practice the Sexual Energy Massage techniques. As stated earlier, the Universal Tao is not responsible for your use or misuse of this practice. The massage techniques are your best protection. Do not neglect them at any time.

PRECAUTIONS AND SUGGESTIONS FOR PRACTICE

The best precaution is common sense. Read this section carefully to fully understand this practice!

Warning: If you know that you already have a blood clot from circumstances that predate this practice, consult a physician about the severity of the problem before attempting Chi Weight Lifting. A blood clot should be fully dissipated for complete safety in these practices. Otherwise, it can dislodge and relocate in a vital area, bringing serious or lethal consequences. A medical consultation should reveal whether or not the Sexual Energy Massage or Chi Weight Lifting techniques can be safely used with an existing blood clot. If not, ask your doctor about options to help circumvent or alleviate the problem. There are medical methods of eliminating blood clots. The Universal Tao is not responsible for your choice, however. Your physician's advice and your internal sensitivities must be your guidelines in such matters.

1. Be sure that the Microcosmic Orbit is clear of any blockages.
2. Be well versed in all of the prerequisites before attempting this practice. Without a degree of mastery of Iron Shirt Chi Kung, which roots the body and draws energy from the earth, a student may not be grounded enough to safely accumulate external energies. Refer to chapter 5 for abbreviated instructions and to *Iron Shirt Chi Kung* (Destiny Books, 2006) for the complete Iron Shirt practice. Without the Six Healing Sounds, the organs may overheat. Without the Microcosmic Orbit meditation, there is no point in doing any practice taught in this system. Trouble would be the only result. Refer to chapter 5 for instructions in the Microcosmic Orbit and the Six Healing Sounds.
3. Men who have not mastered the Sexual Power Lock, and therefore cannot prevent an ejaculation, should not practice Chi Weight Lifting. Practice Healing Love such as Testicle Breathing and Scrotal Compression, given in chapter 1, instead. If you have mastered these techniques, but you lose your seminal fluid accidentally, abstain from Chi Weight Lifting for at least two to three days after the accident. Be prepared to drastically reduce the weight you would normally lift, since chi diminishes with the loss of seminal fluid, making the practice unsafe.

   It is safe to practice Chi Weight Lifting after sex, provided that the seminal fluid is retained. You should still be prepared to reduce the weight, however, if the act of sex drains you in any way.
4. The ancient Taoist masters advised that one abstain from sex for the first one hundred days of this practice. For the best results in the modern world, abstain at least until you have comfortably mastered the lightest weights. Do not try to speed up your progress for this purpose. This is recommended because you must

fully retain your sexual energy before you can safely practice Chi Weight Lifting.

5. Take extra care not to allow the accumulation of too much sexual energy in the head. Headaches, numbness, or discomfort can be alleviated by pressing the tongue to the roof of the mouth and drawing the pressure out of the head, down through the tongue, and into the navel. Spiral the energy, following the same procedures used at the end of the Microcosmic Orbit meditation.

6. Remember that the Scrotal Compression exercise found in chapter 1 is the best way to replenish the sexual energy you are extracting from the testicles. Use this after the Chi Weight Lifting practice.

7. Upon mastering Chi Weight Lifting, the testicles may be drawn into the body after the weights are removed. Do not be alarmed. No harm will come of this, provided that you relax and don't cause yourself any injury through fear or rash action. You may employ the Scrotal Compression technique, but it is not absolutely necessary. The testicles will descend by themselves within a few minutes or, at the most, a few hours.

In ancient times it was considered a priceless asset for a male martial artist to be able to retract his testicles into the body to avoid having them crushed or damaged by an opponent. In spiritual circles, this was a valued practice because the maintenance of Ching Chi could no longer tax the organs and glands if no sperm were produced. (The testicles cannot produce sperm in a retracted state.) Taoist adepts who practice to this end will eventually acquire full access to their internal energy.

Sexual energy transforms into life-force energy, which transforms into spiritual energy. The ability to stop the actual production of sperm or eggs means there is one less transformation for energy to go through, since life-force energy becomes directly available. This should not be taken to mean that such a practice is being advocated but to inform you of its ramifications. The ancient masters saw this as a short-cut to the cultivation of spiritual energy, leaving one with fewer steps to cover on the spiritual path.

8. Never try to lift weights without using the entire groin. The cloth must be tied around the penis and the testicles together. Using the testicles alone defies common sense; however, there are those who can be tempted to try new things without first reading the instructions.

9. Never lift weights with an erection. This can lead to a great deal of pain as the pressure of the weight expands into the already engorged head of the penis. Further, lifting with an erection may create conditions that can lead to blood clots.

10. To help prevent painful slippage of the cloth, tighten the knot at the base of the testicles so that it almost touches the perineum. Try to avoid too much slack around the groin while lifting, but do not cut off circulation.

11. In the beginning stages of practice, you might feel a little pain in the groin or in the abdomen caused by the lifting of the weight. Massage very carefully before and after Chi Weight Lifting, and follow the procedures with caution. The massage should reduce any pain you may experience.

    Once your sexual organs become stronger, the pain will gradually go away. This is not unlike the muscle pain that occurs in normal weight lifting. Some men may experience fever, but there have been no reports of infections of the testes resulting from this practice. You may wish to use only the massage techniques until the pain stops, and then resume lifting.

12. If you feel pain in your internal organs after training, practice the Microcosmic Orbit meditation and the Six Healing Sounds until the pain is gone. The pain may be a sign of overheating, which means that Chi Weight Lifting should be discontinued until the pain subsides. This may also be an indication that your internal organs are not in a healthy condition. If so, practice the less advanced techniques instead of Chi Weight Lifting until you can comfortably lift weights.

13. If you scratch the skin of the sexual organs, clean the area, and allow it to heal before you do this practice. It is best to avoid lifting weights if the groin is hurt. You may apply medications that you have used before, providing that the sexual organs are kept dry. (Hydrogen peroxide is useful for keeping a wound clean and dry.) Avoid using most medications on or around the sensitive tip of the penis.

14. Although it is better to lift less weight for longer periods of time than to lift heavier weights for shorter periods, avoid lifting any weight for more than 60 seconds. You must avoid cutting off the circulation of blood to the testicles.

15. Do not try to outdo yourself or anyone else, because you then stand a good chance of getting hurt. If you feel any strain at all, remove the weight immediately.

16. If you haven't practiced for more than a week, do not return to the same weight you were able to lift before the layoff. Build up again slowly to avoid injuring yourself.

17. When energy is low, and you still choose to practice, spend more time massaging the genitals, and less time hanging the weight.

18. When some people detoxify, diarrhea, nausea, or pain in some of the organs may result as they are cleansed by the process. These are all temporary; however. Chi Weight Lifting (along with the Hitting practice given in *Bone Marrow Nei Kung*) can also initiate some long-term effects that are ultimately good:

    • During the first 100 days of practice, a reduced sex drive may result from the transfer of sexual energy up to the higher centers to heal the organs and glands. Once the body has had a chance to repair itself, the sexual energy will increase greatly, thereby restoring the sex drive.

    • A need to drink more water may result from changes in metabolism.

    • Practice may cause either an increase or loss of appetite, accompanied by exhaustion. This may be part of the rebalancing process that the body goes through as energy is being assimilated.

Some overweight people begin to lose weight; some underweight people find that they are eating more.

- When you practice Chi Weight Lifting you may feel heat, muscle spasms, shakiness, coldness, breezes, or simply an overall "funny" feeling. The body may not yet be adjusted to the increase in chi, or the energy may be fighting diseases in the body, thereby causing such symptoms. Use your own judgment as to whether you should continue the process, but if serious physical problems persist, consult your doctor.

- As certain levels of practice are attained, some people dream profusely. This may be because they are practicing Chi Weight Lifting and Hitting in excess, or they may be hitting too hard. This causes the organs to overheat. Also, if the physical body is too hard and tight, emotions may be locked in the muscles and organs. The Hitting process may release them. Pain felt in the tendons and muscles can cause a great deal of dreaming. The increase in chi, and its fight against diseases of the body, can cause great internal changes, which may also be the source of excessive dreaming.

19. Be especially careful if you suffer from high blood pressure. Concentrate on opening your Microcosmic Orbit. Once it is open and flowing, blood pressure can be reduced and eventually controlled.

20. Do not practice Chi Weight Lifting on a full stomach. Wait at least one hour after a meal before practicing. Also, to keep from losing chi when you have finished exercising, do not eat for one-half hour to an hour.

21. Do not shower right away after practice, especially if you sweat. Allow your body to cool down for a while. You are still absorbing chi at this point; therefore, it is better to avoid washing away external energy.

22. If you have washed before practicing, be sure to dry yourself thoroughly. Otherwise, you may abrade yourself if your skin is still moist when you apply the weight.

23. You may wish to cut your pubic hair short. If it is left long, pain may result if it is pulled during Chi Weight Lifting.

24. Urinate or have a bowel movement before practice. If this is not possible, try to wait one or two hours after practice before fulfilling these functions in order to prevent any loss of accumulated chi. This will give the body time to absorb the chi into the bones, organs, and glands. Collect the energy in the navel.

25. In hot weather, do not drink too much cold water because the body must expend a great deal of internal energy to warm it. This may result in too much cold energy in the heart, which can be harmful.

26. Many people have reported a loss of desire for alcohol, drugs, tobacco, coffee, and tea as a result of the detoxification initiated by Chi Weight Lifting. It is best to avoid these toxic substances in any case, but keep in mind that they will satisfy you less if you detoxify faster than these substances are taken in. The stimulation they offer may not occur if they are forced out of the body before they can affect you.

27. Do not stand on a cold floor during practice. If there is no rug, stand on a towel. A cold floor will draw away your energy.

28. In the early stages, avoid practicing at night, because you may not be able to sleep. When you become proficient, you should be able to practice at any time.

29. Remember that the purpose of your training is to raise your energy levels and to rid your body of toxins. It is *not* to promote violence or foolishness. Do not walk into your local bar and make claims to being "the sexual weight-lifting champion of the Universal Tao." You may find that this particular subject is not well received in certain social atmospheres.

30. Be aware that practices that draw sexual energy into the body can spread any existing venereal infection. Be sure that you are free of such problems before attempting the Sexual Energy Massage or Chi Weight Lifting.

Warning: Be aware of your body's reactions to Chi Weight Lifting. Although this system is known for its many safeguards for avoiding side effects, it is difficult to account for the internal differences in people. *Any* problems that do not appear to be covered in this book must be directed to the Universal Healing Tao. In such cases, Chi Weight Lifting should be discontinued until you are fully aware of your status.

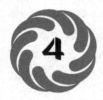

Cleansing, Detox, and Nutrition for Prostate Health

For optimum prostate health, you need to assist the proper functioning of the prostate gland by opening up and cleaning out what are known as the front and back doors of the body. In addition, proper nutrition supports health and strength in every way and following certain nutritional guidelines can be particularly effective in prostate cancer prevention.

THE BACK DOOR

The Colon

The key to the health of the back door, and in many ways the health of the whole body, is how well you eliminate the toxins and built-up debris you have ingested. For the colon—which includes the anus, rectum, and the whole lower abdomen—Taoists highly recommend regular cleansing practices to clear out any buildup of toxins. The most important of these practices are colonics and dry skin brushing; also recommended are solar bathing, rectum cleaning, and a natural-sponge face wash. These cleansing practices are described in more detail below.

In general, breathing deeply and mindfully—by expanding the lower abdominals to draw air in and thus expand the lungs, and then flattening the abdominals to push the used air out of the body—helps to activate and repair all of the body's natural eliminative processes. In this way, any type of aerobic exercise will help elimination by activating the lungs, which then activate their paired organ, the colon. Conversely, when you clean out the back door you will also improve your breathing.

If you have never cleaned out your colon or rectum, and have been building up toxins for twenty or thirty or forty years, you can just imagine what you have in there. You need to cleanse this area of the body just as you do the other end of the body (the mouth and the teeth). As you cleanse the colon you will start to eliminate a lot of excess body fat and acids.

Colonics

Colonics are a method of flushing the colon with water to clear out impacted food waste and debris. There are two main types of colonics— an open-ended type and a closed-end type. The open-ended colonic involves the insertion into the rectum of a thin-tipped hose, which is connected to a container filled with lukewarm water. Other ingredients, known as implants, might be added to the water, including chlorophyll, coffee, garlic, Epsom salts, or a combination of these. A closed-end colonic device is operated by a colon therapist. Its metal insert sends water into the colon and pulls the evacuated debris out.

The process of a colonic is similar to a mouthwash, except that it happens in the colon. You wash the internal skin of the colon and thereby release any blockages. But whereas the closed-end type uses a machine to push water in and flush it back out, the open-ended type relies on gravity and the actual rectal muscles to eliminate the water solution and its accompanying debris. In this book we will be describing methods and practices for open-ended colonics that you can do at home; if you prefer, however, you can have them performed at a professional facility instead (see fig. 4.1 on page 104).

A colonic series consists of one colonic every other day for a week to two weeks. You should do a series every six months to cleanse out your

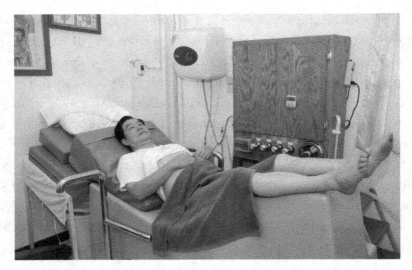

Fig. 4.1. Colonic cleansing at a professional colonic facility

whole body. The only caution is that colonics will draw out from the digestive wall a lot of the natural bacteria that you need to digest food; you will need to include acidophilus supplements so you can culture the bacteria again within the colon.

With an open-ended colonic you will fill up a bucket of water, put it over the toilet to give it gravity, and sit on a special board as you hook tubing up over the toilet.* As you slowly release water from the tip of the bucket tubing into the rectum, you can massage your abdomen and also do light aerobic exercises to help your body eliminate (figs. 4.2 and 4.3).

One of the problems with the colon is that human beings stand upright—unlike other animals, who are on all fours. Because of our upright stance, our bodies have to move waste up the body in the ascending colon, against gravity. This means that someone with deficient chi may become constipated, further exacerbating any unhealthy condition. Once you are cleaning your colon regularly you will start to realize that how you defecate is important. Odors, gas, and even the way you sit become important details of your daily life. If you have a very cleansing

---

*See the resource section at the end of the book for sources of colonic boards, tubing, and other necessary colonic supplies.

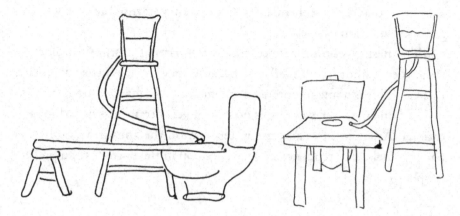

Fig. 4.2. Set-up for an open-ended colonic
that can be self-administered

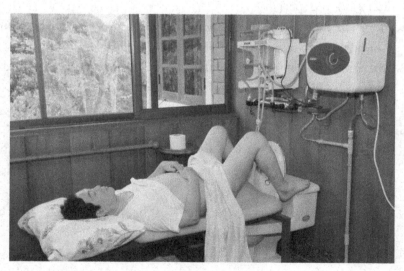

Fig. 4.3. Massaging the abdomen while using a self-operating colonic board

diet that includes a lot of chlorophyll, for instance, there will be no smell at all to defecation, or any gas either. Much of the gas and the smells we associate with our bowels come actually from improper foods that do not agree with the body. It is the horrible combinations of what we put into our bodies—the animal products, the acidic products, the sugars, and starches—that create a chemical reaction as they start to break down; this leads to explosions of gas.

The best position for defecating is a squatting posture. In much of Asia, they do not have toilet seats because they squat on their haunches instead. This is a much more hygienic method because you do not physically sit on anything, so there is no risk of germ transmission. Many traditional Asian cultures also use water to wash the anus instead of toilet paper, which has a tendency to get matted up in the buttocks and prevent proper drying.

 ## Colonic Cleansing

1. Set colonic board hood on toilet and board on stool or use a professional colonic specialist.
2. Hook up tubing to bucket; then fill it with warm water and rinse. Check water release.
3. Insert rectal tip into tube in board hood. Place pad on board and lie on your back on the board with your buttocks on the hood.
4. Apply rectal gel and insert rectal tip into anus.
5. Relax. Release tube clamp. Allow water to flow freely.
6. Massage the left side of your lower abdomen—the descending colon—in an upward direction (against its normal direction of flow) toward the bottom of the ribcage. Work through any tender spots. Continue across the transverse colon just below the ribcage, and then down the right side, which is the ascending colon.
7. When it becomes necessary to evacuate, relieve the bowels by expelling water. Feces will normally bypass the tip without pushing it out.
8. Repeat steps 5–7 a few times until the bucket is empty (about 45 minutes). Do not flush the toilet during the entire colonic. Instead, look at what comes out (it will be black/green feces).
9. To finish, clamp the tube, remove the tip, and slip out from the board. Wash the board; then sit on the toilet to defecate.
10. Clean yourself; then collect energy at your navel point as follows. Starting at the navel, spiral the energy outward in a clockwise direc-

tion, making 36 revolutions. Once you have completed the clockwise revolutions, spiral inward in a counterclockwise direction 24 times, ending and collecting the energy at the navel.

Do two colonics per day for seven days, or one colonic every other day for two weeks.

⚙ Implants

Implants are additives that are placed in the water during a colonic. They can be used to nourish the body and aid cleansing. They can be combined or taken individually.

- Chlorophyll liquid concentrate (½ cup of liquid squeezed from green grass)
- Coffee (2 tablespoons ground coffee simmered in 1 quart of water for 15 minutes, strained and added to bucket)
- Garlic (3 cloves blended and strained into bucket)
- Lemon juice (¼ cup strained into bucket)
- Saline (1 tablespoon of sun-dried sea salt dissolved into bucket)
- Epsom salts (1 tablespoon dissolved into bucket)
- Glycothymoline (8 ounces per 5 gallons of water)
- Acidophilus (1 quarter of bottle into bucket)

After your colonic series ends, eat only whole fruits and vegetables for 2 days. They can be steamed or cooked into soup. Also take acidophilus twice a day for 2 weeks.

Dry Skin Brushing

In Chinese medicine, the skin is often called a "third lung" because of its connection to the lungs and large intestine. For this reason, a colon cleanse also includes opening and cleaning out the pores of the skin with dry skin brushing and solar bathing. Skin brushing should be done on a

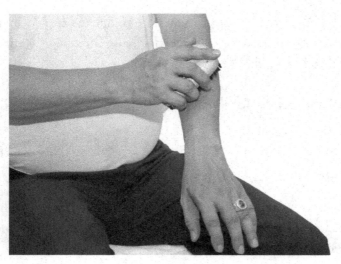

Fig. 4.4. Dry Skin Brushing

regular basis for maintenance, youthfulness, and longevity, and should be included in the periodic colon cleanse (fig. 4.4).

Use a bristle brush or loofah brush before your morning bath and before bed at night. Gently brush with strokes from outer points of the body to the center. The skin should glow with a pink color; it should not turn red. The total process takes about 3 minutes.

1. Do the Inner Smile meditation (see chapter 5 for directions on how to do the Inner Smile meditation).
2. Beginning at the sole of the right foot, brush from sole of foot up the entire leg to the groin. Use short quick strokes or long sweeping strokes toward the heart. Use as many strokes as are needed to brush the front, back, and sides of the leg.
3. Repeat step 2 on the left leg.
4. Brush buttocks, hips, lower back, and abdomen with circular motions.
5. Brush the left arm from the hand up to the shoulder, then circle the left breast. Make sure to brush the top, bottom, and sides of the arm.
6. Repeat step 5 on the right arm and breast.
7. Brush across the upper back, then down the front, back, and sides of the torso. Cover entire skin surface once.

8. Use a softer brush on the face. Begin in the center of the face and stroke outward. Brush down the sides of the face and neck.
9. To finish, jump into the shower and feel a light, tingling sensation over your body.
10. Clean and dry your body, then collect energy at the navel point as follows. Starting at the navel, spiral the energy outward in a clockwise direction, making 36 revolutions. Once you have completed the clockwise revolutions, spiral inward in a counterclockwise direction 24 times, ending and collecting the energy at the navel.

Solar Bathing

Expose your entire body to the open air to absorb vitamin D (fig. 4.5).

1. Use the Inner Smile meditation to smile down to your organs (see chapter 5 for directions).
2. Lie down naked in a secluded area, absorbing fresh air and the sun's rays for 10 minutes on each side.
3. Work up to 30 minutes on each side by adding 5 minutes each day.

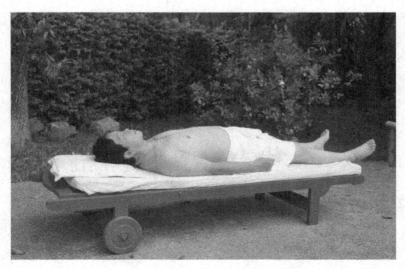

Fig. 4.5. Solar Bathing

4. Collect energy at the navel. Do the Six Healing Sounds. (See chapter 5 for directions on how to practice the Six Healing Sounds.)

◯ Rectum Cleansing

After defecating on the toilet, it's a good time to clean the rectum. Men can also massage the prostate at this time.

You will need the following supplies: a surgical glove or plastic finger cot, castor oil, Dr. Bronner's pure castile soap.

1. While sitting on the toilet after completing your bowel movement, cover your middle finger with a finger cot or surgical glove and insert it into your rectum. Clean out your rectum, massaging the upper roof of the rectum wall. This massage will effectively massage the prostate.
2. Remove your finger, keeping the finger cot on, and apply castor oil. Reinsert the finger into your rectum and clean again. It may take several rounds of cleaning to complete the process, as you are likely to experience a few more bowel movements while you do it.
3. Remove the glove and clean your hands with pure castile soap.

◯ Natural Sponge Face Wash

You can perform this facial wash any time your skin feels tight or dry. When done on a regular basis it can prevent dry skin and signs of aging. You will need a natural sea sponge and cool purified water for this practice.

1. Soak the sea sponge in purified water and gently apply it to your face (fig. 4.6). You can gently clean, rub, and massage your skin.
2. After completing the wash do not dry your face. Instead, allow it to dry naturally, so that your facial skin will absorb the purified water.

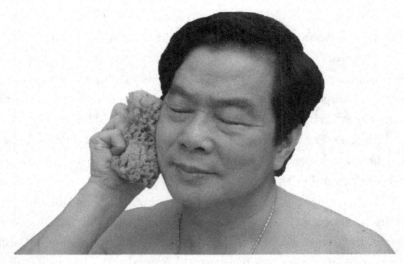

Fig. 4.6. Natural Sponge Face Wash

Cellular Cleansing

While you are doing a colonic cleanse, we suggest you do a cellular cleanse at the same time to improve your results. This cleanse consists of a 7–14-day fast, during which you ingest only vegetable broths and specific herbs and supplements. These supplements will activate the energy and debris in your system, so that they are more easily removed by the colonics.

This cellular cleanse came from natural health pioneer Victor Irons over ninety years ago; it recommends oral bentonite and psyllium for cleansing the colon and taking supplements to strengthen and build up the cells. Together, the supplements—including chlorophyll, digestive enzymes, and essential fatty acids—draw toxins out of individual cells and into the intestinal system, where they can be effectively eliminated. Then psyllium and bentonite help to pull the debris off of the colon walls, which allows you to eliminate this caked up material from your body.

Bentonite is a form of clay that was once blown into the sky by volcanic action, then sifted down to earth, where it collected in layers or veins that can be mined. Its action is due to three things. First, its large and varied mineral content gives it a negative electrical charge, which attracts positively charged particles. In the human body, much of the toxic poisons are positively charged. Second, the minuteness of the particles of bentonite give it a very large surface area in proportion to its volume, thus enabling it to pick up many times its own weight in positively charged particles such as body acid debris. Third, to obtain maximum effectiveness in the human body, it should be in a liquid colloidal gel state. For information on where to buy colloidal bentonite and the other supplements recommended in this cleanse, see the resource section at the end of this book.

Clays have been used as natural medicines for thousands of years. Nutrition pioneer Weston A. Price found it in common use among the Yucatan Indians of Mexico, for instance. When an Indian had a cut, bruise, abrasion, or irritation, he would immediately make a "mudpie" with a certain clay and apply it to the affected area to help it heal. The Yucatan people also took clay internally; when they did not feel "up to par" generally, they would immediately go to this special clay and mix it into a solution with water and drink it. This seemed to relieve whatever symptoms were present, and in a great many cases, these people seemed to live to a ripe old age.

Indigenous people from places as diverse as the Andes, Central Africa, and Australia have also been known to ingest clay. In many cases people regularly dipped their food into clay to prevent a "sick stomach."

The Cellular Cleanse (with Colonics)

This is a liquid fasting cell cleanse that uses bentonite, psyllium, and various supplements for a period of 7–14 days, with a colonic every other day for greatest results. You should eat nothing for the 7–14 days of the cleanse, but you may drink herbal teas or vegetable broths.

Note that you should always consult your physician about your ability to complete this cleanse. If you are able, we recommend that you do this cleanse 2–4 times a year.

You will need the following supplies for this cleanse: a pint jar, apple juice, apple cider vinegar, honey, bentonite, psyllium seed husks, and the supplements listed in the table on page 114. Sources for purchasing these supplements are listed in the resource section. You will also need the colonic supplies listed in the resource section.

The cleanse consists of two drinks mixed separately. Drink them in succession 5 times per day.

First Drink

Place all of the ingredients in jar. Shake for 15 seconds. Drink quickly.

2 ounces apple juice, lemon juice, or lime juice for
flavor
8 ounces pure water
1 tablespoon colloidal bentonite
1 teaspoon psyllium

Second Drink

Place all ingredients in pint jar. Shake, and drink quickly.

10 ounces pure water
1 tablespoon apple cider vinegar or other vinegar
1 teaspoon honey or pure maple syrup

Supplements

Along with the two cleansing drinks you will need to take the supplements 4 times a day on the days specified, as listed in the table on page 114. You should separate the cleansing drinks and the supplements by 1½ hours. For example, if you take the cleansing drinks at 7:00 a.m., you should take the supplements at 8:30.

SUPPLEMENT SCHEDULE (4 TIMES PER DAY)

	Day 1	Day 2	Days 3, 7, 14
Chlorophyll gel tablets	12	18	24
Vitamin C tablets	200mg	200mg	800mg
Pancreatic enzyme tablets	6	6	6
Beet tablets	2	2	2
Dulse tablets	1	1	1
Enzymatic tablets	2	2	2
Niacin tablets	50mg	100mg	200mg
Wheat germ oil tablets	1	1	1

THE FRONT DOOR

The Urinary Tract and Genitals

For the urinary tract, which includes the penis, prostate, testicles, bladder, and kidneys, most of the cleansing practices focus on the kidneys. As the source of sexual energy, the kidneys are a vital energy center that needs to be kept in good health. To help to keep the kidneys clean and in prime condition, Taoists highly recommend herbal teas, vegetable cleanses, and Sexual Energy Massage on a regular basis. These will help to clear out any debris, blockages, and built up toxins from the urinary tract.

Cleansing the Kidneys

The kidneys are extremely delicate, blood-filtering organs that congest easily. Dehydration, poor diet, weak digestion, stress, and an irregular lifestyle can all contribute to the formation of kidney stones. Most kidney grease/crystals/stones, however, are too small to be detected through modern diagnostic technology, including ultrasounds or X-rays. They are often called "silent" stones and do not seem to bother people much. When they grow larger, though, they can cause considerable distress and damage to the kidneys and the rest of the body.

To prevent kidney problems and kidney-related diseases, it is best to eliminate kidney stones before they can cause a crisis. You can easily detect the presence of sand or stones in the kidneys by pulling the skin under your eyes sideways toward the cheekbones. Any irregular bumps, protrusions, red or white pimples, or discoloration of the skin indicates the presence of kidney sand or kidney stones.

 ## Herbal Kidney Cleanse

The following herbs, when taken daily for a period of 20–30 days, can help to dissolve and eliminate all types of kidney stones, including uric acid, oxalic acid, phosphate, and amino acid stones. If you have a history of kidney stones, you may need to repeat this cleanse a few times, at intervals of 6 weeks.

> Marjoram (1 ounce)
> Cat's claw (1 ounce)
> Comfrey root (1 ounce)
> Fennel seed (2 ounces)
> Chicory herb (2 ounces)
> Uva ursi (2 ounces)
> Hydrangea root (2 ounces)
> Gravel root (2 ounces)
> Marshmallow root (2 ounces)
> Goldenrod herb (2 ounces)

Directions

1. Thoroughly mix all the herbs together and put them in an airtight container. You may put them in the refrigerator.
2. Before bedtime, put 3 tablespoons of the herb mixture in 2 cups of water. Cover, and let it sit overnight.

3. The following morning, bring the concoction to a boil; then strain it. (If you forget to soak the herbs in the evening, boil the mixture in the morning and let it simmer for 5 to 10 minutes before straining.)
4. Drink a few sips at a time in 6 to 8 portions throughout the day. This tea does not need to be taken warm or hot, but do not refrigerate it. Also, do not add sugar or sweeteners. Leave at least 1 hour after eating before taking your next sips.
5. Repeat this procedure for 20 days.

If you experience discomfort or stiffness in the area of the lower back, this is because mineral crystals from kidney stones are passing through the ducts of the urinary system. Normally the release is gradual and does not significantly change the color or texture of the urine, but any strong smell or darkening of the urine that occurs during the kidney cleanse indicates a major release of toxins from the kidneys.

Note: Support your kidneys during this cleanse by drinking extra amounts of water, a minimum of 6–8 glasses per day. However, if the urine is a dark yellow color, you will need to drink more than that amount.

Bone Marrow Soup Kidney Cleanse

Make a bone marrow soup with the following ingredients, and drink it on a regular basis to maintain kidney performance and health.

Cracked organic beef bone (knuckles), marrow
   exposed
Seaweed (hijiki or nori)
Garlic
Added vegetables: Carrots, onions, zucchini, celery,
   burdock root, daikon radish

Kidney Tonics

The following preparations tone the kidneys and increase their ability to filter impurities from the blood.

- Cranberry juice (unsweetened) with an equal amount of purified water
- 1 to 2 lemons juiced in purified water

OPTIMUM NUTRITION FOR PROSTATE HEALTH

The three vital functions of food are to rebuild the living tissues, to supply energy, and to preserve a proper medium in which the biochemical processes of the body can take place. To ensure that all three take place, it is important to follow twelve rules of healthful eating.

1. Eat only when hungry and stop before you are full.
2. Maintain proper balance of acid and alkaline and yin and yang.
3. Chew your food well and mix thoroughly with saliva.
4. Refrain from eating when emotionally upset or physically exhausted.
5. Eat food at room temperature.
6. Eat fresh, natural, organic raw and cooked foods daily.
7. Fast or follow an eliminative diet when necessary.
8. Combine food properly.
9. Refrain from close eye work or intense brain work before, during, or after meals.
10. Eat your last meal at least three to four hours before bedtime.
11. Be cheerful and calm at mealtime.
12. Follow the law of moderation.

An elaboration of all twelve keys to good health, along with extensive nutritional guidance for health and longevity, can be found in our book

Cosmic Nutrition (Destiny Books, 2012). Here we focus on maintaining an alkaline-based diet, necessary to achieve the optimum results from the Prostate Chi Kung exercises.

Balancing Acid and Alkaline

In order to grasp the significance of acid and alkaline, we must first understand the meaning of pH, which is a measure of hydrogen ion concentration in blood, urine, and liquids, and is used as symbol to indicate acidity and alkalinity. A pH of 7 (.0000001 gram atom of hydrogen ion per liter) is considered neutral, the measure of pure water. The acid end of the pH scale is from 1 to 7, and 7 to 14 is the alkaline end. In the human body, a slightly alkaline blood and lymph is a requirement for health and long life.

Solvent type foods such as watery fruits, juices, and nonstarchy vegetables are alkaline. The heavier type foods are acid: all proteins, starches, fats, and sugars, that is, all nuts, seeds, cheeses, bread, potatoes, rice, oils, dried and sweet fruit, like dates, raisins, figs, bananas, and so on.

All ripe fruits are alkaline-reacting within the system. These alkalines neutralize the acid poisons, uric acid, and acidosis, which usually come from a high-protein meat diet. In addition, according to Chi Kung master, Jeff Primack, in his book *Conquering Any Disease,* ellagic acid, which is considered to be a cancer inhibitor, is found in forty-six different fruits. Its richest source is raspberries.

Cancer Inhibitors

In *Conquering Any Disease,* Jeff Primack also specifically recommends certain other foods for their support of overall health and cancer prevention:

- Asparagus, which boasts the highest glutathione levels of any food, glutathione being unmatched in its ability to remove poisons from the body.
- Pumpkin seeds, which contain zinc, a mineral necessary for proper prostate functioning.

- *Agaricus blazei,* a mushroom with legendary immune system benefits.
- Black beans aid kidney functioning and sexual disorders.
- Kidney beans are also said to strengthen the kidneys; in addition they are rich in protein and very warming and nourishing.

As explained in the work by Lino Stanchion in his book *Power Eating Program,* for cancer prevention, foods need to be chewed completely for maximum results and benefits. In addition to promoting a more alkaline condition in the body, chewing activates and balances all

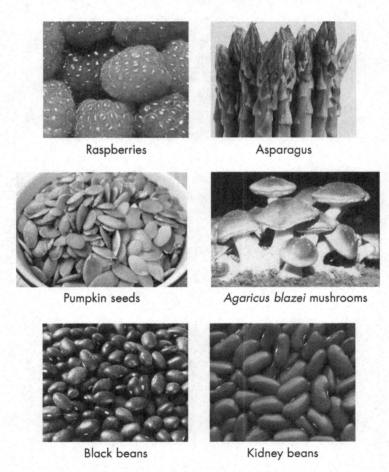

Raspberries   Asparagus

Pumpkin seeds   *Agaricus blazei* mushrooms

Black beans   Kidney beans

Fig. 4.7. Prostate health power foods

the glands, from the pituitary and thyroid to the pancreas, spleen, and gonads.

Another route is that suggested by Primack in *Conquering Any Disease* and *Smoothie Formulas,* in which foods are taken in smoothie form, such as in the Alkalizer Smoothie recipe shown here.

The Alkalizer Smoothie

Blend together:

- 1½ cup distilled water
- 3 stalks of organic celery
- ½ organic cucumber
- ½ lime with pith and seeds
- 1 Fuji apple sliced with skin and seeds
- 3 leaves of Swiss chard
- 1 node of cilantro

Prostate Chi Kung Summary

The exercises and practices in this book are meant to enhance and heal the body's sexual energies through Prostate Chi Kung for the prevention of any type of prostate cancer while rejuvenating your sexual vitality. In addition to the exercises summarized below, your prostate health will be supported by the cosmic detox and nutritional practices detailed in chapter 4.

You should proceed with caution and patience when doing the Prostate Chi Kung practices, allowing the body to respond in a timely manner.

Prostate Chi Kung Daily Practices:

1. Inner Smile
2. Microcosmic Orbit
3. Six Healing Sounds
4. Testicle Breathing
5. Scrotal Compression
6. Iron Shirt Chi Kung
7. Bone Breathing
8. Bone Compression
9. Increasing Chi and Kidney Pressure
10. Power Lock

11. Sexual Energy Massage
12. Chi Weight Lifting

These practices are described here in a condensed format so you can practice them using these pages as guidelines to help you master the formulas of Prostate Chi Kung.

PREPARATION:
INNER SMILE AND MICROCOSMIC ORBIT

The energy from your mother that formed your body entered it through the umbilical cord, then moved from the navel down to the sacrum, then up the spine to the crown (Governing Channel), then down the front of the body (Functional Channel), back to the navel. As long as you are alive your energy moves within this Microcosmic Orbit. Once you become aware of this flowing energy, you can use it to heal any internal energy blockage in your body.

The Microcosmic Orbit meditation is initiated by the practice known as the Inner Smile, which draws positive energy to the internal organs and glands. For both, sit on the edge of a chair with your hands held together and eyes closed. Full descriptions of these practices can be found in *The Inner Smile* (Destiny Books, 2008) and *Healing Love through the Tao* (Destiny Books, 2005).

The Inner Smile

Front Line: The Functional Channel

1. Be aware of smiling cosmic energy in front of you and breathe it into your eyes.
2. Allow smiling energy to enter the point between your eyebrows. Let it flow into your nose and cheeks, and let it lift up the corners of your mouth, bringing your tongue to rest on your palate.
3. Smile down to your neck, throat, thyroid, parathyroid, and thymus (fig. 5.1).

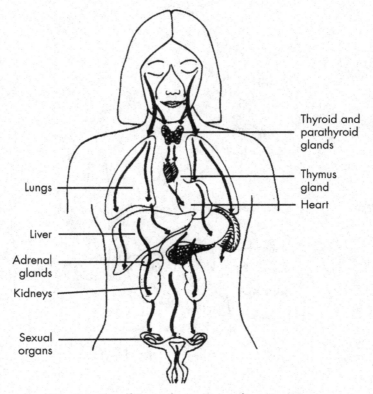

Thyroid and
parathyroid
glands

Thymus
gland

Heart

Lungs

Liver

Adrenal
glands

Kidneys

Sexual
organs

Fig. 5.1. Front line smile: major vital organs

4. Smile into your heart, feeling joy and love spread out from there to the lungs, liver, spleen, pancreas, kidneys, and genitals.

◎ Middle Line:
The Digestive Tract

1. Bring smiling energy into the eyes, then down to the mouth.
2. Swallow saliva as you smile down to your stomach, small intestine (duodenum, jejunum, and ileum), large intestine (ascending colon, transverse colon, and descending colon), rectum, and anus (see fig. 5.2 on page 124).

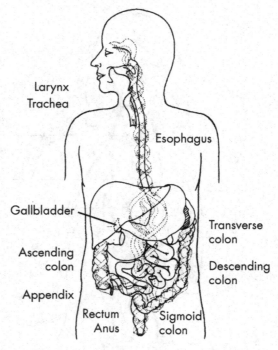

Larynx
Trachea

Esophagus

Gallbladder

Transverse
colon

Ascending
colon

Descending
colon

Appendix

Rectum
Anus

Sigmoid
colon

Fig. 5.2. Middle line smile: digestive tract

🜲 Back Line:
The Governor Channel

1. Smile, and look upward about 3 inches into your mid-eyebrow point and pituitary gland.
2. Direct your smile to the Third Room, the small cavity deep in the center of your brain (fig. 5.3). Feel the room expand and grow with the bright golden light shining through the brain.
3. Smile into the thalamus, pineal gland (Crystal Room), and the left and right sides of the brain.
4. Smile to the midbrain and the brain stem, then to the base of your skull.
5. Smile down to the seven cervical vertebrae, the twelve thoracic vertebrae, the five lumbar vertebrae, then the sacrum and the tailbone.

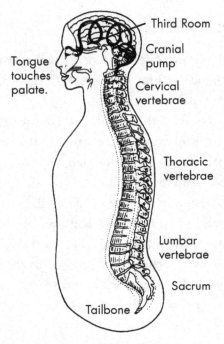

Third Room

Tongue
touches
palate.

Cranial
pump

Cervical
vertebrae

Thoracic
vertebrae

Lumbar
vertebrae

Sacrum

Tailbone

Fig. 5.3. Back line smile: Governor Channel

6. Refresh the loving, soothing smile energy in your eyes, then smile down the front, middle, and back lines in succession. Now do all of them at once, feeling bathed in a cooling waterfall or glowing sunshine of cosmic energy, smiles, joy, and love.

☉ Collect Energy in Navel

1. Gather all the smiling energy in your navel area—about 1½ inches inside your body. Spiral that energy with your mind or your hands from the center point to the outside. (Don't go above the diaphragm or below the pubic bone.)
2. Men spiral clockwise 36 times, then counterclockwise 24 times, returning energy toward the center. Finish by storing energy safely in the navel.

Microcosmic Orbit

1. After smiling down, collect the energy at the navel.
2. With the tongue touching the roof of the mouth, let the energy flow down to the sexual center.
3. Move the energy from the sexual center to the perineum.
4. Draw the energy up from the perineum to the sacrum.
5. Draw the energy up to the Ming Men, opposite the navel.
6. Draw the energy up to the T11 vertebrae.
7. Draw the energy up to the base of the skull.
8. Draw the energy up to the crown and circulate it.
9. Move the energy down from the crown to the mid-eyebrow.
10. Pass the energy down through the tongue to the throat center.
11. Bring the energy down from the throat to the heart center.
12. Bring the energy down to the solar plexus.
13. Bring the energy back to the navel.
14. Circulate the energy through this entire sequence at least 9 or 10 times (fig. 5.4).
15. Collect the energy at the navel. Cover your navel with both palms, left hand over right. Collect and mentally spiral the energy outward from the navel in a clockwise direction, making 36 revolutions. Once you have completed the clockwise revolutions, spiral the energy inward in a counterclockwise direction 24 times, ending and collecting the energy at the navel.

SIX HEALING SOUNDS

The Six Healing Sounds are produced subvocally and correspond to five specific organs: the lungs, kidneys, liver, heart, and spleen. The sixth sound is the "triple warmer," which evenly distributes energy throughout the body. Each sound creates its own energy to enhance and detoxify the internal system. All six sounds and their related postures decelerate the body after practice and remove excess heat accumulated in vital areas. A

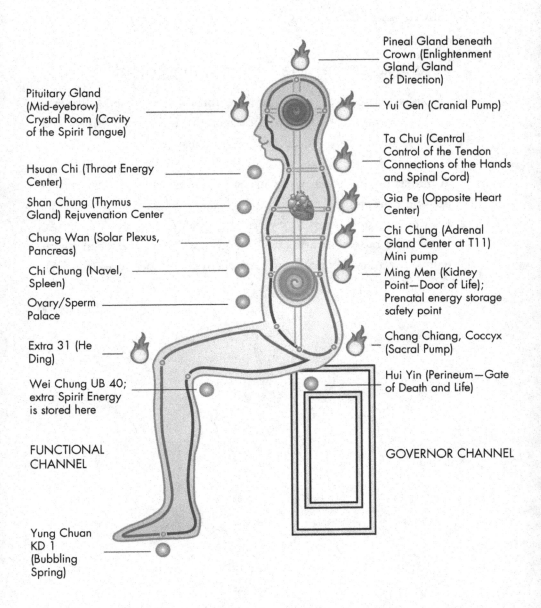

Pineal Gland beneath Crown (Enlightenment Gland, Gland of Direction)

Pituitary Gland (Mid-eyebrow) Crystal Room (Cavity of the Spirit Tongue)

Yui Gen (Cranial Pump)

Ta Chui (Central Control of the Tendon Connections of the Hands and Spinal Cord)

Hsuan Chi (Throat Energy Center)

Shan Chung (Thymus Gland) Rejuvenation Center

Gia Pe (Opposite Heart Center)

Chung Wan (Solar Plexus, Pancreas)

Chi Chung (Adrenal Gland Center at T11) Mini pump

Chi Chung (Navel, Spleen)

Ming Men (Kidney Point—Door of Life); Prenatal energy storage safety point

Ovary/Sperm Palace

Extra 31 (He Ding)

Chang Chiang, Coccyx (Sacral Pump)

Wei Chung UB 40; extra Spirit Energy is stored here

Hui Yin (Perineum—Gate of Death and Life)

FUNCTIONAL CHANNEL

GOVERNOR CHANNEL

Yung Chuan KD 1 (Bubbling Spring)

Fig. 5.4. Energy circulating in the Microcosmic Orbit

full description of this practice can be found in *The Six Healing Sounds* (Destiny Books, 2009).

Lung Exercise: The First Healing Sound

The lungs are associated with the large intestine, the metal element, autumn, dryness, white color, pungent flavor, the nose, sense of smell, and the skin, as well as sadness, grief, courage, and justice.

1. While sitting in a chair with your eyes open, rest your hands—palms up—on your thighs.
2. Breathe in slowly and deeply and bring awareness to your lungs. Inhale and raise your arms until hands are at eye level, then rotate palms inward and continue to raise them above your head (fig. 5.5).

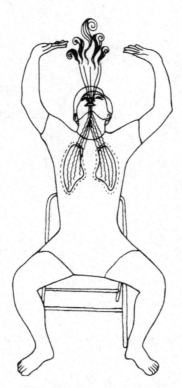

Fig. 5.5. Lung exercise

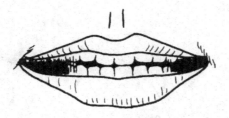

Fig. 5.6. Lungs' sound: sss-s-s-s-s-s

Feel all along the arms into your shoulders, and feel the lungs and chest open.

3. Close teeth and make the lungs' sound: "sss-s-s-s-s-s" slowly and evenly as you exhale (fig. 5.6). Picture the lungs exhaling a dark murky color, excess heat, and sick energy, sadness, sorrow, and grief.

4. Float palms down to lungs and then to your lap, facing up. Breathe in pure white light and the quality of righteousness. Close your eyes and smile to your lungs, imagining that you are still making the lungs' sound. Repeat these steps 3–6 times.

Kidney Exercise: The Second Healing Sound

The kidneys are associated with the urinary bladder, the water element, winter, cold, blue color, salty flavor, ears, hearing, and the bones, as well as fear and gentleness.

1. Breathe in slowly and deeply and bring awareness to your kidneys. Bend forward and clasp your hands together around your knees (see fig. 5.7 on page 130). Pull back on arms, feeling a stretch on your back, over the kidneys. Look up.

2. Round your lips and make the kidneys' sound: "choo-oo-oo-oo," while pulling your mid-abdomen in toward your spine (see fig. 5.8 on page 130). Blow out a dark, murky color along with any excess heat; wet, sick energy; and fear.

3. Breathe in bright blue energy and the quality of gentleness. Separate

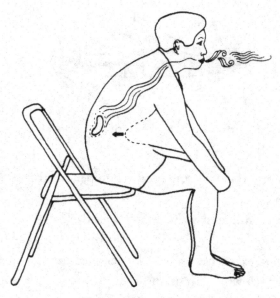

Fig. 5.7. Kidney exercise

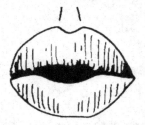

Fig. 5.8. Kidneys' sound: choo-oo-oo-oo

your legs and rest your hands, palms up, on your thighs. Close your eyes and smile to your kidneys, imagining that you are still making the kidneys' sound. Repeat these steps 3–6 times.

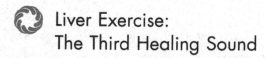 Liver Exercise:
The Third Healing Sound

The liver is associated with the gallbladder, the wood element, spring, moistness, the color green, the sour flavor, the eyes, and eyesight, as well as with anger, aggression, kindness, and forgiveness.

1. Breathe in slowly and deeply, becoming aware of the liver and its connection to the eyes. Beginning with your arms at your sides, palms out, slowly swing your arms up and over your head, following them with your eyes (fig. 5.9). Then interlace your fingers and push palms up toward the ceiling, feeling the stretch through arms and shoulders. Bend slightly to the left.

2. Open your eyes wide and exhale the sound "sh-h-h-h-h-h-h" subvocally (fig. 5.10), while breathing out a dark murky color filled with excess heat and anger.

3. Press the heels of your palms outward as you lower your shoulders, then place your hands in your lap, palms up. Breathe in a bright green energy and its quality of kindness. Let this energy fill your liver. Close your eyes and smile down to your liver. Repeat these steps 3–6 times.

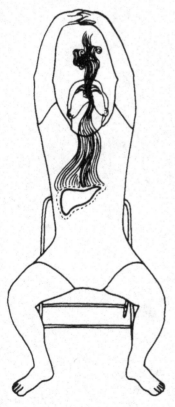

Fig. 5.9. Liver exercise

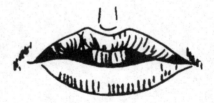

Fig. 5.10. Liver's sound: sh-h-h-h-h-h-h

⟳ Heart Exercise: The Fourth Healing Sound

The heart is associated with the small intestine, the fire element, summer, warmth, the color red, the bitter flavor, the tongue, and speech, as well as with joy, honor, love, creativity, and enthusiasm.

1. Breathe in slowly and deeply while focusing your awareness on your heart. Beginning with palms in your lap, inhale and swing your arms overhead, then clasp fingers together and push palms toward the ceiling, as in the liver exercise (fig. 5.11). This time, bend slightly to the right.

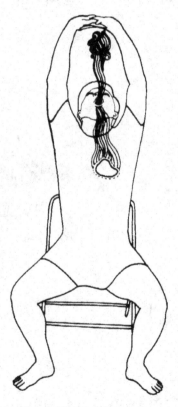

Fig. 5.11. Heart exercise

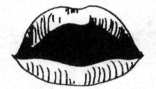

Fig. 5.12. Heart's sound: haw-w-w-w-w-w

2. Open your mouth, round your lips, and exhale the sound "haw-w-w-w-w-w" subvocally (fig. 5.12), while expelling dark murky energy along with any excess heat, impatience, arrogance, or cruelty.
3. Press palms outward and return hands to your lap, with palms facing upward. Breathe in bright red energy along with its qualities of joy, love, and respect. Smile down to your heart. Repeat these steps 3–6 times.

Spleen Exercise: The Fifth Healing Sound

The spleen is associated with the stomach and the pancreas, the earth element, Indian summer, dampness, the sweet flavor, the yellow color, the mouth, and taste, as well as with worry, compassion, balance, and openness.

1. Breathe in slowly and deeply, focusing your awareness on the spleen. Inhale and place the fingers of both hands beneath the left side of the ribcage, just below the sternum (see fig. 5.13 on page 134). Press your fingers inward as you push your middle back outward.
2. Exhale as you round your lips and make the sound of the spleen: "who-o-o-o-o" from your vocal cords (see fig. 5.14 on page 134). Expel any excess heat, dampness, worry, or pity.
3. Breathe a bright yellow light into your spleen, stomach, and pancreas, filling them with fairness, compassion, and centeredness. Lower your hands slowly to your lap, palms up, and smile down to your spleen. Repeat these steps 3–6 times.

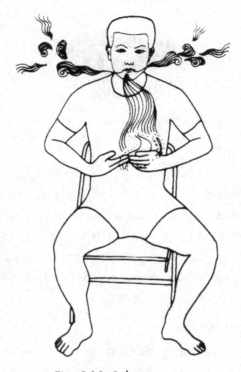

Fig. 5.13. Spleen exercise

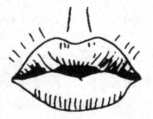

Fig. 5.14. Spleen's sound: who-o-o-o-o

 ## Triple Warmer Exercise:
The Sixth Healing Sound

The triple warmer consists of the upper warmer (hot: includes the brain, neck, thymus, heart, lungs), the middle warmer (warm: includes the liver, stomach, and spleen), and the lower warmer (cool: includes the intestines, kidneys, and genitals).

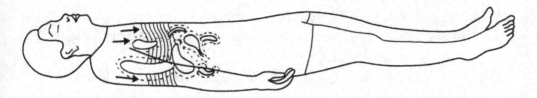

Fig. 5.15. Triple Warmer exercise

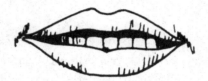

Fig. 5.16. Triple Warmer's sound: hee-e-e-e-e-e

1. Lie on your back, close your eyes, and take a deep breath (fig. 5.15). Inhale fully into all three heaters.
2. Exhale with the sound "hee-e-e-e-e-e" made subvocally (fig. 5.16). Imagine a large roller pressing out your breath from the top of your chest and rolling down toward your lower abdomen. Imagine your chest and abdomen are flat feeling light, bright, and empty.
3. Rest by breathing normally, then repeat these steps 3–6 times.

TESTICLE BREATHING AND SCROTAL COMPRESSION

These two Healing Love practices rechannel sexual energy to heal the internal system. A full description can be found in *Bone Marrow Nei Kung* (Destiny Books, 2006).

 ## Testicle Breathing

1. Sitting: Scrotum hanging free; palms on knees; chin tucked in; head held high.

2. Standing: Hands at sides; feet shoulder-width apart.

3. Lying on your right side: pillow raising head; right fingers in front of right ear with right thumb behind right ear; left hand on left thigh; right leg straight, left leg bent.

4. Tongue to palate; close eyes; be aware of testicles. Inhale slowly through nose and pull testicles up. Hold and exhale slowly, lowering your testicles and feeling cool energy in the scrotum. Repeat 9 times.

5. In turn, inhale and pull up, hold, then exhale and lower, 9 counts each time: to Sperm Palace, sacrum, T11, Jade Pillow at the base of the skull, and crown.

6. At the crown, spiral the energy in your brain 9–36 times clockwise, then 9–36 times counterclockwise. Allow the energy to flow down to the third eye, tongue, throat, heart, solar plexus and the navel. Collect the energy at the navel.

Scrotal Compression

1. Sit on the edge of a chair with testicles hanging loose over the edge or practice in a standing position.

2. Inhale deeply and compress the energy into an imaginary energy (chi) ball at the solar plexus; roll it down to navel, pelvic region, and scrotum.

3. Contract the abdominal muscles downward and pack and compress chi into the scrotum for as long as you can. Squeeze the anus and tighten the perineum to prevent energy loss.

4. While maintaining the compression, keep your tongue pressed against your palate; swallow deeply into the sexual center.

5. Exhale. Take a few quick short breaths by pulling your lower abdomen in and pushing it out (Bellows Breathing) until you can breathe normally. Relax completely.

6. Repeat 3–9 times until the testicles feel warm.

7. Collect energy at the navel and do Bone Breathing.

IRON SHIRT CHI KUNG

The Iron Shirt postures ensure that you have correct structural body alignment, and when they are practiced with the Iron Shirt packing technique, they enable you to build an Iron Shirt body to protect your vital organs. By simply standing and packing in the Iron Shirt postures for five to ten minutes a day, you will root yourself to earth and build a strong body that can live for hundreds of years. Only the first of the several Iron Shirt postures is given here, Embracing the Tree. Full descriptions of all of the postures can be found in *Iron Shirt Chi Kung* (Destiny Books, 2006).

 ## Embracing the Tree

In addition to the packing described below, the Embracing the Tree posture is also used for practicing Bone Breathing and Bone Compression, as well as Chi Weight Lifting (see fig. 5.17 on page 138).

1. Feet shoulder-width apart and the nine points of the feet in contact with the earth.
2. Tilt your sacrum back, round the scapulae, sink the chest, tuck the chin in.
3. Extend your arms as if circling around a tree. Keep your thumbs up and your pinkies down, and the rest of the fingers together.
4. Breathe through the mid-eyebrow point, focusing your eyes on your palms. Feel energy 1½ inches below the navel.

Lower Abdominal Breathing

1. Inhale into the area below the navel. Feel air rush into your lungs as the diaphragm drops. Feel the lower abdomen and perineum bulge on all sides.
2. Exhale forcibly through the nose, feeling a ball rolling up your chest.

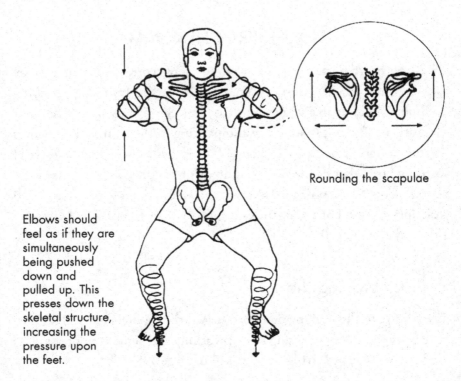

Rounding the scapulae

Elbows should feel as if they are simultaneously being pushed down and pulled up. This presses down the skeletal structure, increasing the pressure upon the feet.

Fig. 5.17. Full Embracing the Tree posture, front view

Sink your sternum and press it into the thymus; at the same time, pull up on your anus and genitals. Flatten abdomen toward spine. Repeat both steps 9–18 times.

♻ Iron Shirt Packing Process, First Stage

During chi packing, your inhalations should be small sips of air; you will inhale many times before you exhale.

1. Contract your perineum and inhale a bit, pulling the genitals up. Inhale again and pull up the left side of the anus. Pack the left kidney and adrenal gland with chi. Inhale a bit more and tighten the right

side of the anus, then pack the right kidney and adrenal gland with chi.

2. Spiral energy at the navel. Circle the energy outward from the navel clockwise 9 times, then counterclockwise 9 times back to the navel center. Spiral your eyes at the same time.

3. With your upper abdomen flat against the spine, inhale into your lower abdomen. Pull up sex organs and the pelvic and urogenital diaphragms, condensing energy into a chi ball in your lower abdomen.

4. Inhale a bit more, pulling the perineum upward as you pack chi into a ball in the perineal area. Hold the breath for as long as is comfortable.

5. Exhale and relax your whole body. Send energy down through legs into the earth.

☯ Iron Shirt Packing Process, Second Stage

1. Press toes and soles of the feet to the floor. Inhale a small breath, pulling earth energy in through the soles. Pull this energy up to the sexual organs, the urogenital and pelvic diaphragms, the left and right sides of the anus, the kidneys, and then into the lower diaphragm. Spiral your eyes and the energy at KD 1 (on the soles of the feet): Spiral 9 times clockwise, from KD 1 outward to a diameter of 3 inches, then spiral 9 times counterclockwise back to KD 1.

2. Inhale, bringing energy from the toes to the knees. Lock the kneecaps and tighten your legs by rotating the knees outward, feel legs like screws rotating into the ground. Energy collects in the knees.

3. Inhale and pull the genitals and anus up, drawing chi from the knees to the buttocks and then to the perineum. Inhale and pack more chi into the perineum. Feel energy moving down into the perineum from the navel, and up into the perineum from the earth through the legs.

4. Exhale and harmonize your breath with abdominal breathing. Relax and smile down to your organs, then practice Bone Breathing.

☯ *Iron Shirt Packing Process, Third Stage*

1. Pack chi into the kidneys, then gather a chi ball at the navel and bring it into the perineum. Push the chi ball into the ground, then bring it up through the soles to the perineum, joining with the energy from the navel that is already there. Harmonize your breathing.

2. Exhale and flatten the abdomen. Inhale a small bit of air while pulling up the back part of the anus to direct the chi into the sacrum. Activate the sacral pump by tucking the sacrum under slightly, without moving your hips.

3. Bring more kidney energy up from KD 1 to the coccyx and sacrum. Inhale, pulling up the anus and packing chi into the kidneys. Now spiral energy at the sacrum: spiral outward 9 times clockwise, to a diameter of 3 inches. Then circle 9 times counterclockwise back to the center of the sacrum. Feel chi collect in the sacrum.

4. Inhale up to T11. Press T11 and the adrenal glands backward, straightening the curve of the low back to further activate the sacral pump. Spiral the energy at T11: circle outward 9 times clockwise to a diameter of 3 inches, then circle 9 times counterclockwise back to the center of T11. Feel sacrum and T11 fuse into one channel.

5. Inhale and pull the chi up from T11 to C7. Push from the sternum to tilt C7 back. Tuck your chin, clench teeth, squeeze the temple bones, and press your tongue to the roof of your mouth (fig. 5.18). When you feel forces pushing at C7, activate the cranial pump. Circle energy at C7: 9 times clockwise out to a diameter of 3 inches, then 9 times inward counterclockwise.

6. Exhale a bit as needed, then inhale and bring the chi up to C1 (Jade Pillow). Spiral energy at C1: outward 9 times clockwise, and inward 9 times counterclockwise, until the chi has developed there.

7. Inhale to crown, to the seat of the pineal gland. Look up between eyebrows to help pull chi to the crown. Circle the chi outward 9 times clockwise, then inward 9 times counterclockwise.

8. Pull up and exhale. Do abdominal breathing to harmonize. Place the

tongue on the roof of the mouth. Bring energy down from the crown to the third eye, then down to the palate, throat, heart center, and solar plexus. Spiral energy at the solar plexus: outward 9 times clockwise, then inward 9 times counterclockwise. Then bring energy to the navel.

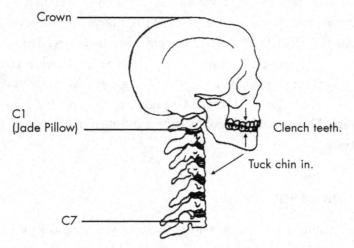

Inhale up to C7. Tilt the neck back and circulate the energy 9 times clockwise and then 9 times counterclockwise. Inhale again, and bring the energy up to C1 at the base of the skull. Circulate 9 times clockwise and 9 times counterclockwise. Inhale, and bring the energy to the crown.

Fig. 5.18. Embracing the Tree, stage three

BONE BREATHING AND BONE COMPRESSION

Bones are extremely porous, and they are always "breathing." The pores allow the passage of oxygen, blood, and nutrition through the bones in the same way a sponge absorbs and releases water. Bone Breathing draws external chi into the bones through the skin, muscles, and tendons. After external energy has been breathed into a particular area, Bone Compression is used to force the combined energies into the bones to burn the fat out of the marrow, thereby assisting in the marrow's regeneration. Step-by-step detailed instructions for the performance of Bone Breathing and Bone Compression, along with further information regarding their health benefits, can be found in *Bone Marrow Nei Kung* (Destiny Books, 2006.)

While Bone Breathing is a mental process used in conjunction with long, soft breath cycles, Bone Compression is a physical process of contracting the muscles, thereby squeezing chi into the bones. This energy is used to complement previously stored sexual energy, which is released into the body through the Sexual Energy Massage or Chi Weight Lifting.

The techniques should initially be practiced from a seated position until you are able to draw the energy while standing in the Embracing the Tree posture.

Bone Breathing

Before beginning the Bone Breathing exercise, you should first be certain that the Microcosmic Orbit is clear of any blockages. Regulate your breathing, then circulate your energy through the Microcosmic Orbit for several cycles.

1. Create a sensation of coolness in the fingers of either hand. Inhale, and draw warm external energies into that hand through the fingers. Apply this to the opposite hand. Exhale, and release the energy.
2. Pull up your genitals slightly as you breathe chi further up into the ulna and radius bones of the lower arm. Practice first on each arm, then on both together. Exhale, and release.
3. Apply the same procedure to the upper arms, drawing chi to the humerus bones. Exhale, and release the energy. Remember to draw energy in with more force with each new inhalation, thereby accessing further points within each limb.
4. Draw chi up through the scapulae and collarbone to reach the C7 point and the cranium but do not leave it there. Either combine it at T11 with the energy drawn from the legs or store it in the navel.

5. Create a sensation of coolness in the toes of either foot. Inhale and draw the warm external energies into that foot through the toes. Apply this to the opposite foot. Exhale, and release the energy.

6. Pull up the genitals slightly as you breathe chi further up into the tibia and fibula bones of the lower legs. If necessary, practice on each leg individually, and then draw chi into both legs together. Exhale, and release.

7. With each breath, draw the chi further up into the femur bones of the upper legs, into the hips, and then to the sacrum. Exhale, but retain the energy you have breathed into these areas.

8. If you choose to combine the procedures for the arms and legs, do not draw the energy to the skull from the arms directly, but instead combine it with the energy from the legs at the center of the spine. First breathe into both hands and feet simultaneously. Inhale chi all the way up to the shoulders and scapulae through the arms, and up to the thigh and hip bones through the legs. Combine this energy at the middle of the spine after it has reached the sacrum and the scapulae from their respective sources. From the center of the spine, move the energy up to the head, and then back down the spine to where the ribs begin. Exhale as needed.

9. Breathe the energy outward through the twelve ribs, encompassing the rib cage from the front to the back, and recombine the chi at the sternum. Breathe into the sternum. Exhale.

Bone Compression

1. Use the same steps as in Bone Breathing, but retain the chi by spiraling it throughout the limbs. Inhale, pulling up the perineum region, then spiral the energy up from the fingers and toes throughout the arms and legs to meet at the center of the spine.

2. Having combined the external energy drawn from both sources at the center of the spine, expand the chi outward through the twelve ribs, spiraling it into the sternum.

3. The body's capacity has been reached when you can no longer spiral

new chi into the arms. Begin to pack the chi, condensing it into the same space as the energy that has been accumulated.

4. Contract the muscles of the hands and arms with each breath. Hold the breath with each contraction.

5. Exhale as you release the contraction. When you release your hold, use your mind to absorb energy into the bones through the pores of the skin. During resting periods, the sensation of drawing in energy through the skin should be felt throughout the body. Bones, muscles, and tendons should begin to feel as though they are wrapped in cotton.

6. After you have practiced for a while, feel the sensation inside your bones. If you have a lot of fat, the feeling will be very hot. This is the fat beginning to melt.

7. It is a good idea to practice with the tongue on the palate because the energy will begin to move through the Microcosmic Orbit; touching the tongue to the roof of the mouth enables the energy to flow in a circle up the spine and down the front of the body.

INCREASING CHI
AND KIDNEY PRESSURE

These two practices, presented in chapter 3, should precede the Power Lock and Chi Weight Lifting. A full description can be found in *Bone Marrow Nei Kung* (Destiny Books, 2006).

Increasing Chi Pressure

1. Place the middle finger of each hand about 1½ inches below the navel.

2. Concentrate on the lower tan tien as you inhale chi into it, expanding the point with the resulting pressure.

Increasing Kidney Pressure

1. Stand in a Horse stance with your feet slightly wider than shoulder width. Rub your hands together until they are warm, and then apply their warmth to the kidneys by placing your energized palms on them from the back.
2. Bend your upper body forward slightly as you inhale, and pull up the left and right sides of the anus as you draw chi up to the kidneys.
3. Exhale, and deflate the kidneys.
4. Follow this sequence up to 36 times, and finish by warming the hands and again placing them on the kidneys.

POWER LOCK

More detail on this practice can be found in chapter 1 of this book, and a full description can be found in *Bone Marrow Nei Kung* (Destiny Books, 2006).

 Power Lock

1. Sit with your feet flat on the floor. Stimulate your jade staff and direct the sexual energy to your testicles and prostate.
2. When you are near orgasm, inhale deeply through the nose. At the same time, clench your jaw and both fists, claw your feet, tighten the cranial pump at the back of your neck, and press your tongue firmly to the roof of your mouth.
3. Inhale again, taking just a short sip of air, drawing up the entire anus and genital region—especially the front part of the perineum. Hold breath then take another short breath. Hold breath again while you contract and pull down the front part of the anus, pulling energy to collect at the perineum.
4. Inhale without exhaling, then clench and pull up your sexual region 9 times, holding energy at the front part of the perineum. Exhale and release all the muscles of the body.

5. Repeat steps 1–3 again, this time continuing to pull the energy up through the perineum and into the coccyx and sacrum. Contract the middle and back parts of the anus as you do this. Arch your sacrum back and outward to activate the sacral pump. Hold the energy here and inhale 3–9 times, creating contractions to pull the energy from the sexual organs. Then exhale and relax.

6. Repeat steps 1–3 again, now drawing the sexual energy up through the perineum and sacrum to T11. Hold the energy at T11, then add the energy from the Sperm Palace by inhaling and contracting 9 times without exhaling. Then exhale and relax, mentally guiding energy from the Sperm Palace to T11.

7. Repeat steps 1–3 again, drawing the energy all the way up to C7. At C7, push the top of the sternum back toward the spine to increase the pumping of energy and to activate the thymus.

8. Repeat the same steps again, this time drawing energy to the Jade Pillow. To activate the cranial pump there, tuck the chin in. Clench your teeth, squeeze the back of your skull, and press your tongue hard against your palate to increase the pumping action.

9. Repeat again, now drawing energy to the crown. Turn your eyes and all senses to the top of the skull and press your tongue firmly to your palate. Practice 9 hard contractions and continue to inhale, each time pulling energy from the Sperm Palace to the crown. With your mind, eyes, and senses, spiral the energy at the crown 9–36 times clockwise, then counterclockwise.

10. Rest and allow the energy to enter your brain. Let extra energy run down the functional channel to the mid-eyebrow point, nose, throat, heart center, solar plexus, and navel.

CLOTH MASSAGE AND SEXUAL ENERGY MASSAGE

The Sexual Energy Massage is preceded by the Cloth Massage to activate Ching Chi. Below are summaries of the practices presented in chapter 2 of this book. A full description of both practices can be found in *Bone Marrow Nei Kung* (Destiny Books, 2006).

 ## Preparation: Cloth Massage

Massage genitals, perineum, and sacrum with a silk cloth. Rotate the cloth around the genitals 36 times clockwise, then 36 times counterclockwise. Feel the testicles loose and full of chi.

 ## Sexual Energy Massage

Rub your hands together briskly to warm them up before performing each of the following steps.

1. Finger Massage of the Testicles: Inhale chi into testicles, and hold one testicle in each hand, with thumbs on top and the fingers underneath. Gently press your thumbs on each testicle, then use the thumbs to massage the whole testicle: 36 times in clockwise circles, then 36 times in counterclockwise circles. Use your fingers to roll the testicles against your thumbs. Roll them back and forth 36 times.

2. Palm Massage of the Testicles: Warm your hands, then cup your testicles in the your left hand while moving your penis aside with the back of the right hand. Lightly press the testicles with both palms, then gently rub them with the left palm—36 times clockwise and 36 times counterclockwise. Warm your hands again, then reverse hand positions and massage with the right palm 36 times in each direction. Draw the energy upward,

3. Duct Elongation Rub: Warm your hands, then cup one testicle in each hand. Use your thumbs and index fingers to gently massage the ducts. Start at the base of the testicles, rubbing the ducts toward the back and the front. Work your way along the ducts toward the body, then reverse direction. Draw energy into the Microcosmic Orbit.

4. Duct-Stretching Massage: Hold the ducts between your thumbs and index fingers. Gently rub your thumbs toward the center, and use

your index fingers to lightly pull the testicles out, stretching the ducts. Repeat 36 times, palm-massaging the testicles in between rounds. Draw the energy upward.

5. Scrotum and Penis Tendon Stretch: Encircle the base of the penis with your thumb and forefinger while your other fingers surround the testicles. Gradually pull the entire groin down toward the tip of the penis as you pull the internal organs up; first, pull straight down with the hand, and then pull down to the left and right in equal counts. Simultaneously pull up the internal organs from the perineum. Hold awhile, then release. Finally, pull the genitals downward in a circular motion 9–36 times clockwise, then counterclockwise. Draw the energy upward.

6. Penis Massage: Use thumbs and index fingers to hold the base of the penis from the sides. Massage the penis along each of three lines, from base to tip and back. Massage each line up and back 36 times.

7. Testicle Tapping: Stand in a wide stance; inhale chi into the testicles, slightly pulling them up, and hold your breath. Clench the teeth while contracting the perineum and anus. Lift your penis out of the way with your left hand, and tap the fingertips of your right hand lightly on the right testicle. Tap in sets of 6, 7, or 9. Exhale, rest, and draw energy up the spine, then change hands and repeat with left testicle.

CHI WEIGHT LIFTING WITH PREPARATORY AND CONCLUDING PRACTICES

We wish to remind our readers that Chi Weight Lifting is included in this text for the documentation of its procedure as a guide for instructors and trained students of the Universal Healing Tao. It is not intended for beginning students. Universal Healing Tao cannot and will not be held responsible for any reader of this book who attempts Chi Weight Lifting without first receiving qualified instruction. A more extensive description can be found in *Bone Marrow Nei Kung* (Destiny Books, 2006).

Preparation for Chi Weight Lifting

To maintain safety, Chi Weight Lifting should always be done after doing the following exercises:

1. Increasing Chi Pressure: Practice from 9 to 81 times.
2. Increasing Kidney Pressure: Practice from 6 to 36 times.
3. Power Lock Exercise: 2 to 3 times up to the crown.
4. Cloth Massage of sexual center, perineum, and sacrum.
5. Sexual Energy Massage:
   a. Finger Massage of the Testicles
   b. Palm Massage of the Testicles
   c. Duct Elongation Rub
   d. Duct-Stretching Massage
   e. Scrotum and Penis Tendon Stretch
   f. Penis Massage
   g. Tapping the Testicles

 ## Chi Weight Lifting

1. Prepare the weight on the floor or a chair.
2. Fold the cloth, and tie it around the penis and testicles. Then tie one end of the cloth to the weight-holding apparatus.
3. Hold the weight or the cloth with your hands while standing up to assume a weight-lifting posture. Test the weight with the index and middle fingers before releasing it.
4. While testing the weight with your fingers, pull up the left and right sides of the anus to the left and right kidneys respectively, and contract the perineum.
5. If it does not feel too heavy, gently release the cloth from the fingers, and hold the weight with the genitals.
6. Swing the weight from 30 to 60 times, inhaling as you pull up with each forward swing. Exhale as the weight moves backward.
7. First lift the weight from each station of the Microcosmic Orbit.

8. Rest as you hold the weight manually, or place it on a raised surface, such as a chair or table top. (You may prefer to remove it while resting, and then attach it again to resume lifting.) Collect the energy in the navel during the rest period.

9. Gently release the weight between your legs once again to lift it with the power of the organs and glands, starting with the kidneys.

10. Lower the weight to the chair or the floor, and untie the cloth from the holding apparatus. Then remove the cloth from the groin.

Concluding Exercises

1. Power Lock Exercise: 2 to 3 times up to the crown.
2. Cloth Massage of the sexual center, perineum, and sacrum.
3. Sexual Energy Massage: Repeat at least 2 or 3 of the Sexual Energy Massage techniques to replenish the circulation of blood in the sexual center and to help dissipate any coagulation, which can lead to blood clots.
4. Use at least 2 or 3 of the Six Healing Sounds, especially the heart and lung sounds. All of them are useful if you have the time to do them.
5. Practice the Microcosmic Orbit meditation for several minutes. In conjunction with this meditation, you can also practice Bone Breathing. Use your mind to absorb the released Ching Chi into the bones.

With these practices of Prostate Chi Kung you now have the opportunity to heal and balance yourself. May the Tao be with you.

# Resources and Recommended Reading

In this section we have listed several sources for the cleansing supplements and colonic supplies that we have recommended in the book, as well as more information on acid and alkaline balance in the diet and recommended nutritional supplements. In addition, a list of books for recommended reading will guide your further study of the topics covered in this book.

CLEANSING SUPPLEMENTS AND COLONIC SUPPLIES

Bernard Jensen International
1255 Linda Vista Drive
San Marcos, CA 92078
Phone: 760-471-9977
Fax: 760-471-9989
E-mail: info@bernardjensen.com
Website: www.bernardjensen.com

Bernard Jensen international carries a wide variety of natural supplements and detoxifying products including colonic boards and supplies. We have listed a few of their supplements below, but see their website for the full range of products.

Niacin

Niacin or nicotinic acid, a water-soluble B-complex vitamin and anti-hyperlipidemic agent, is 3-pyridinecarboxylic acid. It is a white, crystalline powder, sparingly soluble in water. Niacin is essential in energy production at the cellular level. Niacin helps maintain proper metabolic function. Niacin is used for lowering the levels of LDL ("bad") cholesterol or of triglyceride in the blood of certain patients. It may be used in combination with diet or other medicines. It may also be used for other conditions as determined by your doctor. It works by decreasing the amount of a certain protein that is necessary for the formation of cholesterol in the body.

Nova Scotia Dulse (Dulse Tablets)

Nova Scotia Dulse is a sea vegetable that is a natural source of essential vitamins, ions, sea salt, and roughage. Harvested from the cold waters of the North Atlantic this premium dulse is then sun-dried to preserve the natural nutrients. Each tablet provides you with a variety of essential vitamins, minerals, protein, and trace elements the way nature intended. These tablets give you the sodium necessary to assist in moving the waste from the cells in a cellular cleanse.

Vitamin C

This natural source vitamin C tablet contains natural vitamin C derived from dehydrated juice of the acerola berry and wild Spanish orange. These food sources provide the vitamin C complex (i.e., bioflavonoids and other synergistic nutrients), factors not present in supplements that use ascorbic acid (chemical form of vitamin C). This vitamin C has a 100 mg equivalent of ascorbic acid per serving, supplying 110 percent of the Recommended Daily Allowance (RDA). Because vitamin C is constantly being utilized, it should be taken in small repeated doses throughout the day. Chewable tablets are ideal for this purpose, providing easy and rapid absorption of the natural vitamin C complex.

Colema Boards of California, Inc.
P.O. Box 1879
Cottonwood, CA 96022
Toll free: 800-745-2446
Phone: 530-347-5700
Fax: 530-347-2336
E-mail: info@colema.com
Website: www.colema.com

The best source for genuine Colema colonic boards, tubing, and supplies. This company also carries a wide variety of supplements and colonic cleansing products.

V. E. Irons, Inc.
P.O. Box 34710
North Kansas City, MO 64116
Toll free: 800-544-8147
Phone: 816-221-3719
Fax: 816-221-1272
E-mail: info@veirons.com
Website: www.veirons.com

V. E. Irons is home of Vit-Ra-Tox Products and manufacturers of quality whole food supplements since 1946. We have listed several products available from V. E. Irons below, but see their website for the full product line.

Detoxificant (Bentonite)
This substance is a natural and powerful detoxificant derived from bentonite, a mineral-rich volcanic clay. The active detoxifying ingredient is montmorillonite ("mont-mor-ill-o-nite"). Montmorillonite possesses the ability to adsorb about forty times its own weight in positively charged substances present in the alimentary canal. Because montmorillonite has such strong adsorptive properties and is not digested, it tightly binds material to be excreted. It is a perfect accompaniment to the Intestinal Cleanser (see below). Mixed together in juice, this cleansing drink offers

the scrubbing and roughage benefits from soluble and insoluble fiber from psyllium and the detoxification properties of bentonite.

Intestinal Cleanser (Psyllium)

Intestinal Cleanser is a finely ground powder of imported psyllium husk and seed. As it contains primarily fiber and no laxative or herbal stimulants, it can be used on a daily basis to assist normal bowel peristalsis. Psyllium has a hydrophilic (water-loving) action that softens hardened mucus lining the bowel wall, facilitating its elimination. The Intestinal Cleanser and Detoxificant (see above) are ideal companion products to be used together for maximum alimentary canal detoxification.

Fasting Plus (Enzyme Supplement)

Never before has the use of antacids and gastric medication to treat indigestion been so prevalent. These types of drugs block the body's natural digestive processes, but this enzymatic supplement aids the digestion process by providing natural digestive enzymes to break down food and promote assimilation of nutrients. Each tablet contains two layers of digestive enzymes. The outer portion contains pepsin, which digests protein into soluble amino acids, proteases, and peptones. Pepsin is activated by the low pH of the stomach, so people suspected of gastric acid deficiency would benefit from it. The inner portion of the tablet becomes activated in the small intestine and contains natural digestive agents: bovine bile salts that promote absorption of lipids and activate pancreatic lipase (a fat-digesting enzyme), and the pancreatic substances amylase (for starch) and proteases (for protein), plus tyrosine, chymotrypsin, and other proteolytic enzymes. Because the inner portion is intended to work in the intestine, the tablets should be swallowed whole.

GreenLife (Chlorophyll Gel Capsules)

GreenLife is a 100 percent vegetable food containing 92 percent dried extracted juices of organically grown cereal grasses: barley, oats, rye, and wheat (no chemical fertilizers or insecticides are used); and 8 percent papain, beets, and sea kelp. The grasses are cut at the young, rapidly growing stage, when the maximum nutrition is in the blade. GreenLife is a concentrated product, retaining its natural balance as a complete all-food supplement. It is nontoxic in any consumable amount and helps balance nutritional deficiencies resulting from consumption of devitalized and processed foods.

Pro-Gest (Vegetarian Pancreatic Enzymes)

The active ingredient in Pro-Gest is papain, which is derived from the papaya fruit. Papain is a natural proteolytic enzyme that breaks down proteins and supports a healthy digestive process. Other ingredients include papaya seed meal, Russian black radish, and betaine hydrochloride in a base of dried juice from organically grown beets—the same powder used for Whole Beet Plant Juice Tablets (see below). The betaine hydrochloride acts to supplement the natural hydrochloric acid in the stomach.

Wheat Germ Oil/Flaxseed Oil

The wheat germ oil capsules contain 73 percent wheat germ oil, an excellent source of the natural vitamin E complex; and 27 percent flaxseed oil, a rich source of unsaturated, essential fatty acids including: alpha linolenic acid, omega-6, and omega-3. Vitamin E is an essential dietary component that is necessary for antioxidant activity in membranes. It regenerates other cellular antioxidants (i.e., selenium and glutathione) after they become oxidized. The essential fatty acids also must be obtained in the diet and are precursors for many hormones and metabolically active compounds. The natural vitamin E in our foods is destroyed during cooking and processing due to heat, light, air, and freezing. Grains lose up to 80 percent of their vitamin E content when milled. Commercially processed vegetable oils are low in vitamin E. It has become quite clear that there is a need for natural vitamin E supplementation in our modern diets.

Whole Beet Plant Juice Tablets

The beets used for this product are organically grown. The whole beet (leaves, stems, and root) is juiced, and the extract is vacuum dried at low temperature to retain maximum quantities of the enzymes, vitamins, and mineral factors. Unlike inorganic sources of iron, the body assimilates iron from the beetroot very easily, because iron is found in an organic complex. Beets also contain potassium, magnesium, phosphorous, calcium, sulfur, iodine, vitamins, and many trace minerals.

PH BALANCED DIET

Website: www.thealkalinediet.org
Provides extensive information about acid/alkaline balance, food lists, and resources for further information.

Website: www.trans4mind.com/nutrition/pH.html
Includes a how-to on urine and saliva testing, food charts, and a look at the science behind acid/alkaline food chemistry.

RECOMMENDED READING

Chia, Mantak. *The Alchemy of Sexual Energy*. Rochester, Vt.: Destiny Books, 2009.
———. *Basic Practices of the Universal Healing Tao*. Rochester, Vt.: Destiny Books, 2013.
———. *Bone Marrow Nei Kung*. Rochester, Vt.: Destiny Books, 2006.
———. *Chi Self-Massage*. Rochester, Vt.: Destiny Books, 2006.
———. *Cosmic Detox*. Rochester, Vt.: Destiny Books, 2011.
———. *Cosmic Nutrition*. Rochester, Vt.: Destiny Books, 2012.
———. *Healing Love through the Tao*. Rochester, Vt.: Destiny Books, 2005.
———. *The Inner Smile*. Rochester, Vt.: Destiny Books, 2008.
———. *Iron Shirt Chi Kung*. Rochester, Vt.: Destiny Books, 2006.
———. *Sexual Reflexology*. Rochester, Vt.: Destiny Books, 2003.
———. *The Six Healing Sounds*. Rochester, Vt.: Destiny Books, 2009.
———. *Wisdom Chi Kung*. Rochester, Vt.: Destiny Books, 2008.
Primack, Jeff. *Conquering Any Disease*. Sunny Isles Beach, Florida: Press On Qi Productions, 2008.
———. *Smoothie Formulas*. Sunny Isles Beach, Florida: Press On Qi Productions, 2008.
Stanchion, Lino. *Power Eating Program*. Asheville, North Carolina: Healthy Products, 1989.

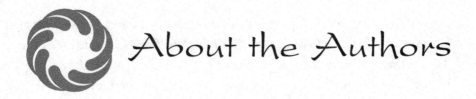 About the Authors

MANTAK CHIA

Mantak Chia has been studying the Taoist approach to life since childhood. His mastery of this ancient knowledge, enhanced by his study of other disciplines, has resulted in the development of the Universal Healing Tao system, which is now being taught throughout the world.

Mantak Chia was born in Thailand to Chinese parents in 1944. When he was six years old, he learned from Buddhist monks how to sit and "still the mind." While in grammar school he learned traditional Thai boxing, and he soon went on to acquire considerable skill in aikido, yoga, and Tai Chi. His studies of the Taoist way of life began in earnest when he was a student in Hong Kong, ultimately leading to his mastery of a wide variety of esoteric disciplines, with the guidance of several masters, including Master I Yun, Master Meugi, Master Cheng Yao Lun, and Master Pan Yu. To better understand the mechanisms behind healing energy, he also studied Western anatomy and medical sciences.

Master Chia has taught his system of healing and energizing practices to tens of thousands of students and trained more than two thousand instructors and practitioners throughout the world. He has established centers for Taoist study and training in many countries around the globe. In June of 1990, he was honored by the International Congress of Chinese Medicine and Qi Gong (Chi Kung), which named him the Qi Gong Master of the Year.

WILLIAM U. WEI

Born after World War II, growing up in the Midwest area of the United States, and trained in Catholicism, William Wei became a student of the Tao and started studying under Master Mantak Chia in the early 1980s. In the later 1980s he became a senior instructor of the Universal Healing Tao, specializing in one-on-one training. In the early 1990s William Wei moved to Tao Garden, Thailand, and assisted Master Mantak Chia in building Tao Garden Taoist Training Center. For six years William traveled to over thirty countries, teaching with Master Mantak Chia and serving as marketing and construction coordinator for the Tao Garden. Upon completion of Tao Garden in December 2000, he became project manager for all the Universal Tao Publications and products. With the purchase of a mountain with four waterfalls in southern Oregon, USA, in the late 1990s, William Wei is presently completing a Taoist Mountain Sanctuary for personal cultivation, higher-level practices, and ascension. William Wei is the coauthor with Master Chia of *Sexual Reflexology, Living in the Tao,* and the Taoist poetry book of 366 daily poems, *Emerald River,* which expresses the feeling, essence, and stillness of the Tao. William U. Wei, also known as Wei Tzu, is a pen name for this instructor so the instructor can remain anonymous and can continue to become a blade of grass in a field of grass.

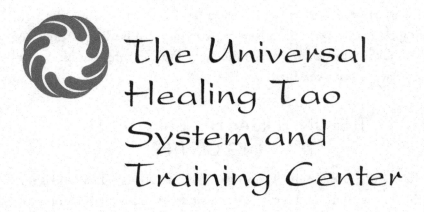

The Universal Healing Tao System and Training Center

THE UNIVERSAL HEALING TAO SYSTEM

The ultimate goal of Taoist practice is to transcend physical boundaries through the development of the soul and the spirit within the human. That is also the guiding principle behind the Universal Healing Tao, a practical system of self-development that enables individuals to complete the harmonious evolution of their physical, mental, and spiritual bodies. Through a series of ancient Chinese meditative and internal energy exercises, the practitioner learns to increase physical energy, release tension, improve health, practice self-defense, and gain the ability to heal him- or herself and others. In the process of creating a solid foundation of health and well-being in the physical body, the practitioner also creates the basis for developing his or her spiritual potential by learning to tap in to the natural energies of the sun, moon, earth, stars, and other environmental forces.

The Universal Healing Tao practices are derived from ancient techniques rooted in the processes of nature. They have been gathered and integrated into a coherent, accessible system for well-being that works directly with the life force, or chi, that flows through the meridian system of the body.

Master Chia has spent years developing and perfecting techniques for teaching these traditional practices to students around the world through ongoing classes, workshops, private instruction, and healing sessions, as well as books and video and audio products. Further information can be obtained at www.universal-tao.com.

THE UNIVERSAL HEALING TAO TRAINING CENTER

The Tao Garden Resort and Training Center in northern Thailand is the home of Master Chia and serves as the worldwide headquarters for Universal Healing Tao activities. This integrated wellness, holistic health, and training center is situated on eighty acres surrounded by the beautiful Himalayan foothills near the historic walled city of Chiang Mai. The serene setting includes flower and herb gardens ideal for meditation, open-air pavilions for practicing Chi Kung, and a health and fitness spa. The center offers classes year round, as well as summer and winter retreats. It can accommodate two hundred students, and group leasing can be arranged. For information on courses, books, products, and other Universal Tao resources, see below.

Universal Healing Tao Center
274 Moo 7, Laung Nua, Doi Saket, Chiang Mai, 50220, Thailand
Tel: (66)(53) 921-200
E-mail: universaltao@universal-tao.com
Web site: www.universal-tao.com

For information on retreats and the health spa, contact:

Tao Garden Health Spa and Resort
E-mail: reservations@tao-garden.com
Web site: www.tao-garden.com

Good Chi • Good Heart • Good Intention

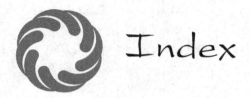 Index

Page numbers in *italics* refer to illustrations.

BOOKS OF RELATED INTEREST

Healing Love through the Tao
Cultivating Female Sexual Energy
by Mantak Chia

Chi Kung for Women's Health and Sexual Vitality
A Handbook of Simple Exercises and Techniques
by Mantak Chia and William U. Wei

Sexual Reflexology
Activating the Taoist Points of Love
by Mantak Chia and William U. Wei

Karsai Nei Tsang
Therapeutic Massage for the Sexual Organs
by Mantak Chia

The Alchemy of Sexual Energy
Connecting to the Universe from Within
by Mantak Chia

Taoist Foreplay
Love Meridians and Pressure Points
by Mantak Chia and Kris Deva North

Healing Light of the Tao
Foundational Practices to Awaken Chi Energy
by Mantak Chia

Chi Self-Massage
The Taoist Way of Rejuvenation
by Mantak Chia

INNER TRADITIONS • BEAR & COMPANY
P.O. Box 388
Rochester, VT 05767
1-800-246-8648
www.InnerTraditions.com

Or contact your local bookseller